Your
Asthma-Free
Child

Your Asthma-Free Child

The Revolutionary 7-Step Breath of Life Program

DR. RICHARD N. FIRSHEIN

AVERY
a member of Penguin Putnam Inc.
New York

Every effort has been made to ensure that the information contained in this book is complete and accurate. However, neither the publisher nor the author is engaged in rendering professional advice or services to the individual reader. The ideas, procedures, and suggestions contained in this book are not intended as a substitute for consulting with your physician. All matters regarding health require medical supervision. Neither the author nor the publisher shall be liable or responsible for any loss, injury, or damage allegedly arising from any information or suggestion in this book. The opinions expressed in this book represent the personal views of the author and not of the publisher.

While the author has made every effort to provide accurate telephone numbers and Internet addresses at the time of publication, neither the publisher nor the author assumes any responsibility for errors, or for changes that occur after publication.

Most Avery books are available at special quantity discounts for bulk purchase for sales promotions, premiums, fund-raising, and educational needs. Special books or book excerpts also can be created to fit specific needs. For details, write Putnam Special Markets, 375 Hudson Street, New York, NY 10014.

a member of
Penguin Putnam Inc.
375 Hudson Street
New York, NY 10014
www.penguinputnam.com

Copyright © 2002 Richard N. Firshein, D.O.
All rights reserved. This book, or parts thereof,
may not be reproduced in any form without permission.
Published simultaneously in Canada

Library of Congress Cataloging-in-Publication Data

Firshein, Richard N.
Your asthma-free child : the revolutionary 7-step breath of
life program / Richard N. Firshein.
p. cm.
Includes bibliographical references and index.
ISBN 1-58333-142-5
1. Asthma in children. 2. Asthma in children—
Alternative treatment. I. Title
RJ436.A68F54   2002   2002025375
618.92'238—dc21

Printed in the United States of America
1   3   5   7   9   10   8   6   4   2

Book design by Stephanie Huntwork

To asthmatic children
and their parents throughout the world

acknowledgments

I would like to give special thanks to the following people: to Delia Marshall for her wholehearted support and creative clarity; to my incredible agent, Kris Dahl at ICM, for her wonderful guidance throughout the years; to Maggie Canon and the staff at Mighty Wors; to Kristen Jennings at Avery for her care and enthusiasm.

Sincere gratitude to Paul Sorvino, a truly noble soul, for his friendship and dedication to helping asthmatic children.

Special thanks also to my parents, Sylvia and Michael Firshein, for their courage, love and inspiration; to Mary Angela Lauricella for assisting with the research for this book; to the many dedicated people who have contributed to the success of the Breath of Life program; to my staff for understanding the importance of taking care of one patient at a time.

My deepest appreciation to Marcia, who has brought so much beauty and peace into my life, and without whose love I could not have written this book.

contents

introduction

We are on the threshold of a new era in the treatment of asthma. Each day, as scientists study everything from nutrition to the human genome, we gain a better understanding of asthma and other diseases. We know much more about what causes asthma, how to treat symptoms, and how to prevent attacks from happening in the first place. We have access to new medications that are more effective and less toxic than drugs of yesterday. We have discovered that a natural, holistic approach can have a profound effect on a chronic disease such as asthma. Parents can now rest easy knowing that asthma doesn't have to be the threat to a child's life that it once was.

I know from personal experience how far we've come. I've been asthmatic all my life. While my childhood was wonderful, it seemed that illness was always around the corner. I remember lying in my bedroom with my inhaler, pumping medicine into my lungs. Many nights as a child I was hunched over a vaporizer with a towel covering my head, hoping that the steam would loosen up my chest. I was frequently sick with upper-respiratory infections, and it seemed as if I was constantly on antibiotics.

I periodically had to contend with the side effects of some very strong drugs, such as epinephrine and Tedral. A popular drug at the time, Tedral is a combination of three medications—*ephedrine,* a stimulant to open up airways, *phenobarbitol,* which calms down the side effects of the ephedrine, and *theophylline.* While I was taking Tedral, I was alternately wired and sleepy, and I often had the odd feeling of being jittery and exhausted at the same time.

Fortunately, as I grew older, new drugs came out that seemed to help considerably. They were the first generation of bronchodilator sprays, called *beta-agonists.* All through my teenage years, as long as I kept my trusty sprays in my pocket, I was pretty much okay.

Then, in my late twenties, as a physician already in practice, I became ill again. But this time it was different. The sprays and other medications that I had come to rely on simply didn't work. It was a total shock. I hadn't even conceived of this possibility. I went straight from the emergency room to intensive care and was put on seven drugs a day just to survive. It was at this point that I almost died of an asthma attack.

As I lay there in the hospital bed, I kept thinking that there had to be a better way. This was the turning point in my life. When I recovered, I began my journey toward true healing by researching all the possible ways to treat asthma. I read thousands of articles. I attended conferences and interviewed leading physicians in the areas of preventive and alternative medicine. Against the advice of just about everyone, I began a program focused on natural remedies and began building up my immune system. I slowly weaned myself off drugs. Today I have never felt better. I rarely need to take any asthma drugs and am virtually asthma-free.

As I look back on my childhood, I can see why my asthma was so bad. We simply didn't know what we know now. No one understood the role of mold, dust-mites, and chemicals like formaldehyde in causing asthma. Doctors had only a hazy idea of what was going on inside the body of an asthmatic person and didn't realize that asthma can cause complications that last a lifetime.

My body endured repeated attacks that had a cumulative effect on my lungs and overall health. No one knew I had food allergies when I was young, and one of my earliest childhood memories is of eating a peanut and immediately becoming violently ill. After that, I knew enough to avoid peanuts but couldn't possibly have known that peanuts and other common allergens like soy products are in many processed and junk foods. And like every other kid growing up in the '60s, I ate my fair share of candy and junk food.

While we had an inkling that air pollution was a problem for asthmatics, no one had ever even heard of *dust-mites,* microscopic critters that live in bedding, upholstered furniture, and carpeting. Airborne mite droppings are a common cause of asthma attacks and must be methodically eliminated from an asthmatic person's house. We also didn't know that dust is another problem for asthmatics. The heating ducts in our house were never cleaned, which meant dust and debris just kept recirculating. My symptoms would increase every fall, but no one made the connection to our heating system. Even if we had, there was no such thing as a company that cleaned ducts in those days.

School was worse. There was a general lack of awareness about the toxins that were in nearly every room in the school. Fumes from the various cleaning solutions were generously swiped over every hallway as if polio itself were lurking in the corners. Chalk dust and coal dust from the coal-fired furnace permeated the air. I remember one year sitting near a covered pail in the corner that contained asbestos blankets, which were to be used to suffocate fires. While the blankets didn't pose an immediate threat, it was an example of the naive way in which dangerous compounds were handled, whether it was asbestos, lead paint, ammonia, bleach, or coal dust.

I now suspect that the drugs I had been taking all those years were probably masking the underlying causes of my asthma, promoting further damage.

Your child doesn't have to live like this. We know a lot more about asthma than when I was a kid in the '60s. I have been studying and treating asthma for more than a decade, and through personal experience and research into all facets of natural approaches to health, I have developed a comprehensive holistic program called Breath of Life. Within six weeks of starting my program, almost all my patients are able to breathe better, have increased confidence, and enjoy a better quality of life. Many of my patients significantly reduce their medications, and some get off drugs altogether. Virtually all of the patients on my Breath of Life program are in control of their asthma.

In 1996 I wrote a book, *Reversing Asthma* (Warner Books), to introduce my Breath of Life asthma-prevention program to the millions of people around the world—both adults and children—who suffer from asthma. As more and more parents asked for guidance about implementing my program, however, I realized that children have very special needs, not the least of which is for parents to play a crucial role in their recovery. Over the past several years, I adapted and perfected my Breath of Life program for kids and their families.

This book describes this very same kid-friendly Breath of Life program that I use in my practice. It offers parents a clear, proactive, health-building anti-asthma regimen that will help reduce your child's asthma symptoms and greatly improve his or her health and quality of life.

Of course, having a child with asthma presents parents with a unique challenge. The variables with asthma are limitless, from what causes it to how to prevent it. In addition to all your other parenting duties, you have to think of so many things that don't come naturally. What are the safe alternatives to toxic cleaning supplies? How do I get my kid to stop craving sodas and Popsicles? What is the best air filter? Where can I find out more about hidden food allergies?

Identifying the particular reason your child suffers an attack can take some persistent detective work. I once treated Todd, a thirty-eight-year-old architect from Iowa, and his eight-year-old son Jason. A few weeks before their first visit, Todd had picked up Jason from his after-school program in the family's brand-new SUV. As they excitedly drove home, they tested all the gadgets, including the radio, the ergonomic drink cups, and the automatic seat controls. They put on the air conditioner full blast, thrilled that it cooled the car in minutes flat, and thought nothing of the slightly odd odor coming from the vents. Unfortunately, that odor was from an anti-mold chemical that many manufacturers routinely spray into the AC units of new cars. Both Jason and his father unwittingly inhaled the chemical all the way home, and both subsequently suffered acute asthma attacks. Eventually they were able to trace their symptoms to the unusual smell coming from the AC vents in their new car.

Breath of Life is a step-by-step program that will enable you to cope with your child's asthma in a coherent, methodical manner. While it does require time and commitment, it is vastly preferable to a childhood of medications, or doing nothing. Just by starting now, you are already boosting your chances for successfully reducing or curing your child's asthma. Early intervention—while your child's body is resilient and responsive with lungs that are still growing—can prevent permanent damage. Moreover, early diagnosis and treatment can stop a cascade of negative psychological effects. When not treated effectively, asthma can negatively shape a child's personality, setting up patterns of frustration and hopelessness that persist across a lifetime. Children can become distrustful of their environment and even of their families when nothing seems to help.

The Breath of Life program gives you the tools to break this cycle of fear. It enables you to give your child the precious gift of health. You will help your asthmatic child to enjoy life more, to play sports freely, to go outside whenever he or she wants, to spend more time with friends. You will also create a healing partnership between you and your asthmatic child. This partnership can lessen the psychological stress a family endures when a child has asthma and encourage your child to move toward an asthma-free life. A healthy child means a healthy family.

chapter one

Get with the Program

The Breath of Life program is a holistic approach that focuses on natural therapies for asthma. It's a step-by-step program that can reduce your child's vulnerability to asthma, increase his self-confidence, and improve his quality of life. Ideally, you will help your child incorporate this program into every aspect of his life.

The program can be broken down into seven parts. First, you will learn about the many potential allergens in your home that could be a trigger for your child's asthma and discover the most effective ways to rid your home of these toxins. Next, a chapter on diet and food allergies explains how to wean your child off unhealthy or allergic foods and to replace them with those that help her grow strong and fend off asthma episodes.

A chapter on medications follows. Asthma drugs are an important part of an overall program toward recovery, and parents should have a basic understanding of the risks and benefits of the most common medications prescribed for children. Often parents assume that because I'm a doctor who practices alternative medicine, I want all children to stop using medications. This is not the case. My focus is to reduce or possibly even eliminate the need for medications by treating the underlying disorder through natural remedies. By following the Breath of Life program, your child should have fewer hospitalizations and a reduced need for asthma drugs. Occasionally, however, drugs are necessary, and this chapter will enable you to make informed decisions about medicating your child.

The next element of the Breath of Life program focuses on nutritional supplements, including a discussion in Chapter 6 of the scientific research that supports the use of these supplements for asthmatic children. In Chapter 7, I explain how to teach your child breathing exercises. These exercises can help her to both breathe easier and relax voluntarily in the face of the panic that can accompany asthmatic episodes. Next, a chapter on visualization techniques that even young children can learn that may help your child offset the stress of asthma. The last part of the program, discussed in Chapter 9, is to help your family cope with the frustrations that can come with asthma.

How can I be so confident that my Breath of Life program works? First, it has worked for the many children I've treated in my practice. But my program has also been put to the acid test. A few years ago, as I started to notice how well all the kids in my care were doing, I mentioned my success to several other asthma doctors. I told them I'm getting the kids off junk food, getting their parents to clean up their environments, training the kids in breathing and visualization techniques—and getting results. My colleagues responded skeptically, claiming that the children's medications were probably responsible for the success of the program.

I took this as a challenge. If I couldn't even convince doctors, how could I spread the word to the millions of parents and children out there who deal with asthma? I needed undeniable proof that this program works, that kids will follow it and get better.

Not too far from where I work in New York City, in the borough of the Bronx, is a school with one of the highest rates of asthma in the country. At the time, the kids at this school were leading lives reminiscent of my childhood—taking lots of medications, eating a lot of junk food, breathing polluted air—completely unaware of alternative ways to deal with asthma. I decided to bring my Breath of Life program to this school. In short, I was putting my program to the toughest test possible.

One doctor told me it was a waste of my time. And, indeed, it was very time-consuming to get started. It took a great deal of effort to coordinate materials, parents, teachers, and the administration.

Finally, with the unwavering commitment of one of the teachers, the school principal, the Paul Sorvino Foundation, and my office staff, I was able to teach the Breath of Life Holistic Asthma Prevention Program to asthmatic second- and third-graders. The program was taught as an educational supplement to the kids' current care, and they were advised to continue their medications and their relationships with their doctors.

The result? According to the principal of the school, almost all of the 150 kids who enrolled in the program improved dramatically. All *peak-flow meter readings* (a standard measure of breathing capacity) steadily increased. School attendance of the students involved went up an average of 65 percent, with one asthma sufferer receiving his class's attendance award. Parents and children reported less need for medication. Parents and teachers noticed an increase in self-confidence, concentration, and sense of well-being in all the kids. Children who previously reported multiple emergency-room visits no longer needed to go to the hospital. One child was even able to teach her mother breathing exercises that averted an emergency-room visit when the mother had an attack in the middle of the night.

I was surprised by how willing to participate in the program the kids were, and by how much fun they had with the breathing exercises. I was repeatedly amazed to witness a classroom full of children lying quietly on mats, peacefully meditating or visualizing, without any of the usual giggling and whispering. In fact, the program was so popular that children without asthma were clamoring to be included. I will never forget the graduation ceremonies; parents, teachers, principals were in attendance, as were the deputy mayor of New York and representatives from the Bronx borough president's office. The kids could hardly contain themselves, running around the stage beforehand, smiling, and shouting. It was impossible not to notice that these kids were behaving in a distinctly asthma-free manner.

The program was considered so successful that Paul Sorvino and I were honored by the American Medical Association and presented with an award by former surgeon general C. Everett Koop. We were even asked to expand the program into other New York City schools, and the Sorvino Foundation is currently raising money so we can do just that.

There is every reason to believe that your child will enjoy the same success with the Breath of Life program. For one thing, he has one of the most powerful asthma-fighting weapons in his corner—You! A team approach will hasten your child's road to recovery and help him realize he is not alone. You will all come to know that you have control over asthma. As a supportive parent, you can provide a learning, caring environment to make healing possible. You can also help make necessary lifestyle changes a lot easier. If you work as a team through each step of the Breath of Life program, you will both come to know that you have control over asthma.

You will also develop a deeper sense of trust with your child. I recently saw Colin, a four-year-old preschooler who is just beginning to recover from a bout of asthma. He was animated as we went through the exam, chattering about how much he liked doing his breathing exercises with his mom. I couldn't help but notice the joint sense of accomplishment between Colin and his mother, and the beautiful sense of trust that had developed.

This unique program is designed to build that type of trust, to allow parents and children to work together, proactively and effectively, to reverse this condition.

chapter two

Why My Child?

hat causes asthma? No one knows for certain. We've learned
a lot in the past few years—it is such a complex condition, for
instance, that at least sixteen separate genes are involved in
asthma—but ignorance has long shrouded the disease. Until the mid-
twentieth century, asthma was thought to be psychosomatic, caused by
a childhood trauma or, some people speculated, by a dysfunctional relationship between mother and child. There was even a hospital where
asthmatic children would be sent for months at a time so they could recover away from home. Of course, while asthma can cause terrific psychological distress, there is no doubt that it is a chronic physiological condition.

WHAT IS ASTHMA?

A couple of decades ago, asthma attacks were thought to be brought on
by constricted airways in the lungs, which in turn make it difficult to

breathe. At the time, asthma was thought to be easily treated. This led to the use and eventual overuse of certain medications, such as bronchodilators and adrenaline-like drugs, that targeted tightened air passages only. Then researchers discovered that asthma is characterized not only by constricted airways but also by excess mucus production and inflammation of the tissues in the lungs and tubes leading to the lungs. This led to the use of newer anti-inflammatory medicines, such as inhaled steroids and Singulair. Added to this mix is one often overlooked aspect of asthma: muscle fatigue. After days or even weeks of trying to breathe in enough air, a deep muscle fatigue can set in around the shoulders and neck, making breathing during an attack even more difficult. It is the interrelationship of these four factors that makes asthma so complex.

When a healthy person inhales, she enlists the diaphragm, a powerful muscle that sits underneath the lungs, to draw in air. The air is filtered and humidified through the nose or mouth, then passed down the windpipe into tubes called the *bronchi,* which then lead into *bronchioles,* or smaller tubes that travel into the lungs. The bronchioles, in turn, deliver the air to millions of tiny air sacs called *alveoli,* which reside deep in the lungs. The alveoli passively expand and contract as oxygen is delivered to the bloodstream and carbon dioxide is sent back to the lungs to be exhaled. In a healthy person, it is a perfectly regulated process, efficient no matter whether one is running, eating, or sleeping.

This process goes awry in asthmatics. When your child tries to breathe during an attack, her respiratory function is compromised. First, the airways constrict. Next, a powerful inflammatory reaction may occur, which activates inflammatory cells such as eosinophils, mast cells, and macrophages. These, in turn, recruit other inflammatory messengers. As tissues in and around the lung become irritated and inflamed, the muscles surrounding the bronchi tighten. *Goblet cells* then secrete mucus, which can clog airways and further irritate the already raw and inflamed tissue. The end result is the common symptoms of asthma:

wheezing, shortness of breath, coughing, phlegm, and tightness in the chest. This complex process is known as the *inflammatory cascade*. Researchers now know that repeated attacks can cause permanent lung damage in some people.

Doctors have broken asthma down into four loosely defined categories:

- **Mild Intermittent:** Symptoms occur less than two times a week, nighttime symptoms occur less than two times per month, episodes are brief and of varying intensity, and in between episodes the patient is fine.
- **Mild Persistent:** Symptoms occur more than two times per week but less than one time per day, nighttime symptoms occur more than two times per month, and physical activity is occasionally impaired.
- **Moderate Persistent:** The patient has daily symptoms and uses sprays daily; episodes that affect activity occur more than twice a week and may last for several days, and nighttime symptoms occur more than one time per week.
- **Severe Persistent:** The patient has continual symptoms, frequent exacerbations and nighttime symptoms, and limited physical activity. Some doctors use terms such as *cough-variant asthma,* where coughing is the only symptom.

Remember that this is a guideline only, and few patients fit neatly into any of these categories. Also remember that all these terms are part of the same spectrum. While the diagnoses may sound unusual, the treatments remain largely the same.

It's important not to confuse symptoms with the disease. One of the biggest problems with asthma is that symptoms don't always tell the whole story. A child may have mild intermittent symptoms, but her underlying inflammation could be serious—much worse than the symptoms lead you to believe. A common misperception is that just because the symptoms are gone for a week, a month, or even a year, the underlying condition is gone. It can take a long time for a child's lungs to heal completely.

Studies have revealed that lung inflammation persists even after symptoms are gone. Scientists have compared the lung tissue of people who died of an acute asthma attack to the lung tissue of asymptomatic asthmatics who died of other causes and found that their lungs look remarkably similar. But there's a lot that we still don't know about asthma. A child may seem fine one day and end up in the emergency room the next.

Still, having an understanding of these broadly defined categories will help you and your doctor deal with each phase of your child's asthma and regulate the treatment as needed.

WHY IS ASTHMA ON THE RISE?

A century ago, asthma was rare. Now it is anything but. Asthma is one of the few chronic diseases on the rise; its incidence has soared by 73 percent since 1982. Nearly 17 million people have asthma, including 5 million children. It is the leading cause of childhood illness, hospitalization, and death in America. Asthmatic youngsters under age fifteen are hospitalized nearly 160,000 times a year and stay more than three days, on average. The asthma death rate nearly doubled from 1980 to 1993 among five- to twenty-four-year-olds. Each year more than 5,500 people die needlessly from asthma.

Asthma cuts across all class and race lines, affects boys and girls, and can last a lifetime. It is slightly more prevalent in African-American and Hispanic children, who also experience more severe disability than do other children. The cost to our country is staggering. Almost $2 billion a year is spent to treat pediatric asthma. Parents with asthmatic children lose $1 billion a year by staying home to care for their children.

There is a growing list of theories as to why asthma has been increasing at such a frightening pace; these include overzealous immunization programs, junk-food diets, and antibiotic overuse. There's even speculation that we're just too clean. Last year a study from the *New England Journal of Medicine* suggested that day-care kids have lower rates of asthma because they are exposed to more viruses and bacteria. This repeated exposure exercises and strengthens the immune system by forcing children's bodies to respond earlier in life to common infectious organisms. But while some exposure to natural inoculation is reasonable, parents of asthmatic children need to exercise appropriate caution. Other research has suggested that colds are the most common trigger of asthma in winter and spring, so sitting your child next to a kid who is in the throes of a viral illness may be unwise.

Many researchers put the blame for the rise in asthma rates squarely on sick air, both indoors and out. Except for the skin, the lungs are the only organ that is constantly exposed to the outside environment. The global rise in respiratory illnesses in the industrialized world could well be attributed to the sick air we are increasingly forced to breathe. Children in industrialized countries suffer dramatically higher rates of asthma than do children in rural and poor countries. The gap ranges from 2 percent of children in China to 30 percent in certain parts of Britain and Australia.

Researchers at Johns Hopkins University recently reported that the increase in microscopic soot particles is likely to be a significant cause of asthma and other illnesses. These particles are so small that they evade our bodies' natural filters and become embedded deep in the lungs. A group of scientists recently warned Congress that global warming would contribute to a rise in greenhouse gases that exacerbate respiratory ill-nesses, including asthma.

In addition, our houses are sealed tight, leaving us to breathe air filled with secondary smoke, dust, dust-mites, and fumes from cleaning solvents, paints, and wall coverings. Carpets that were once woven from wool are now made of vapor-emitting synthetics. Formaldehyde-laced plywood, used in virtually every building and renovation, emits gases for up to a year after being installed.

WHAT CAUSES ASTHMA?

Certain people seem to be susceptible to asthma. These include those with a genetic predisposition: Asthmatic children tend to have parents who are asthmatic or allergic. Other risk factors include low birth weight, infection with organisms such as *Chlamydia pneumoniae* or respiratory syncytial virus, and living in an urban environment.

Early exposure to common allergens such as dust-mite and cock-roach droppings appears to increase the risk for asthma. Exposure to these toxins during the first few years of life, the theory goes, can *sensitize* the body, making the immune system respond ever more frantically to further exposures.

Many asthma sufferers, however, don't fall into any of these risk categories, and we simply don't know why they get asthma.

WHAT TRIGGERS AN ASTHMA ATTACK?

Fortunately, over the past several years asthma researchers have identified various *triggers* that can lead to an attack. Unfortunately, there are many of them. Some asthmatics have chemical sensitivities to pollutants such as ammonia or formaldehyde. Colds and respiratory infections can also be triggers. Many cases of asthma can be traced back to a severe cold or respiratory infection. Often this is one of the first times that parents notice a change in their child's condition.

About 20 percent of all asthma episodes are *exercise-induced*. We don't know precisely why exercise-induced asthma occurs. Our best guess is that during intense exercise, fluid from the lining of the lungs is lost faster than it can be replaced. Exercise also places an increased demand on the lungs for antioxidants such as vitamin C or E. One intriguing study showed that kids who took vitamin C before exercise had fewer attacks and better lung function than those who didn't.

Other people get *cold-induced* asthma, and, again, the theory is that lung fluid is depleted too rapidly when you breathe in cold, dry winter air. This can be compounded by the fact that many asthmatic children have sinus conditions, so they're not able to breathe through their nose. The nose can increase humidity in the air to about 99 percent, whereas when we breathe through our mouth, the humidity in the air may reach only 60 to 70 percent.

Asthma can also be caused by *reflux,* a condition where the highly acidic contents of the stomach leak through a small valve into the esophagus. This can cause extreme irritation to the throat, pharynx, nasal passages, and lungs.

It should come as no surprise that living with a person who smokes greatly increases the risk of asthma and asthma attacks. Parents who smoke should stop.

Perhaps the most common trigger for asthma, however, is allergies. Studies have shown that people with the highest levels of allergy antibodies in their blood have the worst asthma. Let's say your child breathes in some pollen to which he or she is allergic. That pollen contains antigens or proteins that link up with IgE antibodies in the skin or bloodstream. This combination acts like a key that unlocks certain cells in the immune system called *mast cells,* which burst open and release their contents. The mast cells contain histamines, which promote many of the typical allergic responses, such as red and watery eyes, rash, nasal congestion, and wheezing. Histamines then provoke other inflammatory chemicals within the body.

The most common allergic triggers include cockroach, mouse, and dust-mite droppings; mold spores, pollens, and pet dander; and foods such as nuts and soy.

Many times an asthma trigger isn't easy to identify. I recently saw four-year-old Hugo, who had just suffered an asthma attack after eating chocolate cake at his birthday party. Hugo's parents were perplexed because it was the same cake, from the same bakery, as last year's. Hugo's dad, Peter, knew that Hugo was allergic to peanuts, which was why he took care to serve a peanut-free cake. Hugo loved chocolate, and Peter was worried that his son had developed an allergy to chocolate. Hugo's parents did not relish the idea of banning it from his life. Peter went back to the bakery to see if there was any change in the ingredients in the cake. The bakery said no. The parents then talked to several of the people at the party and discovered that Hugo had eaten some plain M&M's at his party. When they got ahold of an M&M package, they read the ingredients, and sure enough, printed right on the package was "may contain traces of peanut." They then discovered that the chocolate morsels that the baker used in the cake had the same peanut caution on the package (chocolate candy, by the way, can contain many potential allergens, including soy, corn syrup, lecithin, milk, and the cocoa itself).

Now Hugo can eat chocolate or cocoa, as long as it passes muster with his parents. His mother usually uses just cocoa to bake cakes or to make chocolate syrup for ice cream or chocolate milk. It took some doing, but these parents did isolate the trigger for that particular asthma attack. One of the primary goals of the Breath of Life asthma program is to help you isolate the asthma triggers that wreak havoc with your child's immune system. Many triggers will be obvious; others will require the process of elimination. Your doctor can assist you by doing allergy tests, which are helpful for most children. These allergy tests are less accurate for children under the age of two, however, because their immune systems are not yet fully developed. In any case, many parents find it helpful to keep a careful journal of symptoms to see if a pattern emerges. If a child wakes up in the morning with asthma and has frequent nighttime episodes, for example, perhaps dust-mites in his or her bedding is the reason. If he or she is sick shortly after eating, allergy or reflux could be the cause.

WILL THERE EVER BE A CURE FOR ASTHMA?

We can only hope so. But first we need to treat asthma like the epidemic it is. We need large, scientifically sound studies that thoroughly investigate some of the preliminary findings mentioned above. Rather than just dosing our kids with more and more drugs, we need to provide a prudent plan that allows every child to breathe cleaner air and encourages children to eat healthy foods.

As it stands now, we have a lot of tantalizing information that indicates that diet may play a role, that cleaning up your environment inside and out helps, that one drug has fewer side effects than another, that mind-body and breathing exercises yield concrete benefits, and that nutritional supplements can reduce underlying inflammation. New government proposals aim to cut pollution from trucks and buses 90 percent over the next ten years. The National Institutes of Health have significantly stepped up research into asthma and allergies. Mainstream medical journals are now looking at the role of free-radical damage and asthma. Asthma is being studied at the cellular and genetic levels. Finally, it seems, asthma is getting the attention it deserves.

In the meantime, you have the power to change the course of your child's asthma. With the Breath of Life program, you can follow a coherent plan that combines increased knowledge about the pathology of asthma with the mounting evidence supporting new and alternative approaches to prevent asthma in your child.

chapter three

Clearing the Air

Purifying the air your child breathes at home may be the most underestimated weapon in preventing attacks. The Environmental Protection Agency (EPA) has listed indoor pollution as one of the top environmental threats Americans face today. It's easy to see why. The typical house, especially new ones, are caulked and insulated and filled with particleboard, paints, and synthetic carpets that emit toxic formaldehyde fumes. Pools of water from leaks around sinks and basements become breeding grounds for bacteria and mold. Pets and pests leave droppings and dander. Heating and air-conditioning systems recirculate dust and dust-mites. Meanwhile, the house is doused weekly with a whole panoply of cleaning chemicals and pesticides.

Study after study suggests that if we all breathed cleaner air at home, we would have many fewer children with asthma. Researchers at Johns Hopkins found that mouse urine and dander are major overlooked allergens, and having mice in the house significantly increases the risk of asthma in children. The number of hours that an asthmatic child is exposed to dust-mites in her home has been shown to correspond with the severity of asthma symptoms. A study of 2,500 Finnish children found a strong correlation between plastic wall materials in schools and homes (most wallpaper contains plastics and glues that produce chemical vapors) and an increase in coughing, shortness of breath, and mucus production. A 1996 study of inner-city children in New York found that they had double the risk of asthma at least partly because their air was polluted with allergens such as mice and cockroach droppings.

Allergy testing, in fact, is probably one of the most important steps in asthma treatment and diagnosis. My book *Reversing Asthma* has a detailed list of most of the possible environmental allergens your child may be exposed to, including trees, grass, molds, and dander from feathers. While some of these may not apply to your child, most asthmatic children should be tested for some of the more common allergens discussed below (see Chapter 4 for more on allergy testing and how the tests are performed).

Unfortunately, the air in your yard or at your child's school may also be a factor contributing to your child's asthma. Nearly 50,000 chemicals are currently in use in the United States, leaching into our water, soil, and air. The National Resources Defense Council estimates that Americans drive 150 million cars and nearly 50 million buses and trucks. Ultrafine particles from this oil and diesel exhaust are so tiny that they can be inhaled deeply into the lungs. Vehicle exhaust also contains toxic chemicals such as formaldehyde, benzene, and carbon monoxide (a poisonous gas that passes immediately from the lungs to the body and blocks the ability of the red blood cells to carry oxygen).

Excess ozone also contributes to air pollution. Ozone in the upper atmosphere is critical in protecting the earth from the sun, but at street level it can be toxic. Ground-level ozone is created by the combination of greenhouse gases, oxygen, and sunlight. While the EPA revised ozone standards to protect children in 1997, 27 million children under age thirteen still live in areas where ozone levels fail to meet these standards. Other airborne chemicals that can irritate the lungs include sulfuric acid, sulfur dioxide, and nitrogen dioxide, all by-products of modern industry. In cities, waste incinerators produce carcinogenic compounds and toxic heavy metals.

Many studies have shown that all this air pollution can increase the chances of developing respiratory infections. Short-term exposure to many of these chemicals can severely impair lung function, and chronic exposure can cause permanent damage. Not only does soot-filled air cause free-radical damage to our lungs, it can also sensitize our bodies to other allergens. A Canadian study found that when asthma patients were challenged with "safe levels" of ozone, they became twice as sensitive to ragweed and grass. Exposure to toxins can also weaken a child's immune system, which means she is more likely to come down with a cold or a virus, which can then lead to asthma.

On top of all this, children may be more susceptible to polluted air because they breathe more air relative to their body weight than do adults. They spend more time outdoors and they're more active, which increases the amount of oxygen and pollution that they inhale. Some children's lungs become a tinderbox waiting for a spark, as they exhibit more and more symptoms until they suffer a full-blown asthma attack.

Of course, there's not much you can do about air pollution at the moment, except keep your child indoors on high-ozone or smog-alert days. Over the long term, you may find it worthwhile to agitate for cleaner air by pressuring your elected officials and nearby corporations to reduce the pollutants spewing into our atmosphere.

One thing you can do right now is follow the Breath of Life steps outlined below to make sure the air your child breathes at home is as toxin-free as possible. The key is to identify and remove the most common triggers for asthma around your home.

Sometimes this is all that is needed. A few years ago I met with Sally, a mother of two young daughters, Alexis and Brianna. She was at her wit's end. Both her daughters had recently started to suffer from severe allergies and asthma. After she told me about her home, it became clear what the problem was: The house had recently been renovated and was filled with dust. She had also bought a lot of new furniture that emitted an unpleasant chemical odor.

It was hard to know where to begin, but we finally settled on the girls' bedroom. Sally bought air purifiers with high-efficiency particulate arresting (HEPA) and charcoal filters for both girls' rooms and methodically did everything she could to remove dust-mite exposure. In six weeks, the girls' chronic coughs and runny noses disappeared, and they were both finally sleeping through the night. A couple of months later, they were feeling so much better that they even started to reduce their medications. Sally's only complaint to me was that no one had previously addressed the triggers that were provoking asthma in her daughters.

I know that a search-and-destroy mission for invisible allergens can be a daunting task, especially for today's busy family. I once saw a lovely young family who lived in a modest house in New Jersey. Diane was a hardworking nurse who worked four twelve-hour shifts a week. Her four-year-old daughter, Chelsea, had allergic symptoms and constant ear infections in addition to asthma. I did some very simple allergy testing and found that Chelsea was allergic to dust-mites. With some quick adjustments, we were able to solve the problem.

The most important change they made was the simplest: putting protective covers on all the mattresses and pillows and removing old carpeting from the girl's bedroom. This caused Chelsea's symptoms to clear up at night, but she was still having problems during the day. Then I discovered that the house had one additional problem: forced-air heat that was drawing air from the basement. Diane couldn't remember if or when the ducts had last been cleaned, so I suggested she hire a service to come over and give the heating system a thorough cleaning. After the workmen did the job and were packing up to go, Diane asked the fore-man if he'd found anything in the ducts. "You don't want to know," he replied. She pressed him, and all he would say was that every house he'd ever worked on had ducts loaded with dust, mouse droppings, and dead bugs. On my advice, Diane also had an electrostatic air filter attached to her furnace. Cleaning up the heating system seemed to do the trick, and soon Chelsea's daytime symptoms disappeared.

As I have explained to Diane and other parents in my practice, the Breath of Life program helps you identify each potential problem area, make appropriate changes, and then move on to the next. It often takes less time than you would think. Sometimes even just keeping your child's bedroom allergen-free can prevent serious attacks, according to a new study out from Johns Hopkins University. Occasionally it's difficult to accept that certain changes have to be made, especially those involv-ing a beloved family pet or wonderful new carpeting. But once you start to see your child get healthier, you realize that the sacrifice is a small price to pay.

GET READY FOR SOME DETECTIVE WORK

Did your child wake up with the sniffles this morning? Is his wheeze worse in the spring? Are his eyes red when he comes home from school? Do his allergies get better in the winter and peak in the spring? All of these are clues that may help you determine exactly what is triggering al-lergy and asthma attacks in your child.

After you've filled out the Homesick Syndrome Questionnaire on page 28, you should walk around your home looking for any potential triggers to eliminate. What kind of heat do you have? Forced air? Where is it being drawn from? Are there any watermarks or discolored patches on the walls, especially in the bathrooms? Is there water in the basement? Have your air filters been cleaned? Has anything changed recently? New carpeting? Renovations? Each question leads to further questions. Think about where your child spends her time—home, classroom, day care, or school—and ask the same questions.

Once you've identified possible sources of allergies, you need to eliminate them. Fortunately, there's a brave new world of allergy products to help you. Owing to the fact that our air quality is perilously close to unacceptable, companies have rolled out some high-tech gadgets that can detect and reduce both the natural and man-made allergens in our air. I have had great success with many, and I provide a list of recommended sources on my Web site (www.drcity.com).

The sooner you do this, the better. Expectant parents with a family history of allergies or asthma will want to set up (and maintain) a nursery that is trigger-free. While there is no guarantee that cleaning up your home will end your child's asthma, doing so can certainly reduce the severity of the problem, resulting in fewer trips to the hospital and a reduced need for medications.

THE MOST COMMON CULPRITS THAT MAKE YOUR CHILD'S AIR *SICK*

Dust Mites

Perhaps the number-one enemy for most asthmatics are dust mites, and most houses are home to millions of them. Dust mites are microscopic tick-shaped parasites that live primarily in places we want them least. Their favorite food is flakes from human skin, and they thrive in warm, humid environments. Basically, where you spend most of your time is where you'll find dust mites—in mattresses, pillows, carpeting, curtains, upholstered furniture, and stuffed toys. Bedding, with its constant source of human skin, is especially attractive to dust mites.

✢ Homesick Syndrome Questionnaire ✢

Here is a list of questions I routinely ask new patients. Add up all the points that apply to get a general sense of how many potential allergens are in your home. If you score from 3 to 5, you'll probably have to make only minor changes to your home environment. A score of 6 to 8 indicates the need for a thorough environmental evaluation. A score of 9 to 11 requires immediate changes, and a score of 12 or above means your home is so toxic, it could well be the sole source of your child's asthma.

1. Do you notice increased symptoms when your child is at home? *3 points*
2. Does he or she feel ill when doors and windows are closed in the winter? *1 point*
3. Does your child feel sick at night or upon awakening? *1 point*
4. Do symptoms disappear or improve when your child leaves home? *1 point*
5. Have you recently purchased new carpeting? Drapes? Furniture? Cabinets or bookcases? A gas appliance, furnace, or stove? Has pressboard, particleboard, or plywood been used in a recent renovation? *½ point for each*
6. Do you dry-clean your drapes and/or clothes? *1 point*
7. If you have a carpet, is it cleaned regularly? *If no, 1 point*
8. Do you store large amounts of newspaper? Cardboard? Cleaning products? Pest-control products? *½ point for each*
9. Do you have any pets? *2 points*
10. Have you recently used cleaning solvents, wood strippers,

varnish, stains, paints, or glues in any part of your home, or during any remodeling? *2 points*

11. Do you have forced-air heat or central air conditioning? *2 points*

12. If so, is the air for your heat or air-conditioning system being drawn from the basement? *1 point*

13. Are there any water stains or discolored patches on the walls of the bathroom or other rooms? *1 point for each room*

14. Do you have water in your basement? *2 points*

15. If you have air filters, have they recently been cleaned? *If not, 1 point*

16. Do you have a problem with pests such as mice or cockroaches? *2 points*

17. Does anyone smoke in your house? *5 points*

Female mites lay up to fifty eggs a day, and each mite eliminates waste about twenty times a day. It is these mite droppings that cause allergy symptoms. They cling to dust, become airborne, and are inhaled by anyone within breathing distance. Even after you destroy the mites themselves, their droppings can remain in your home for a long time.

Dozens of studies have shown that dust-mites produce allergic reactions, and certainly a large number of my patients have dust-mite allergy. If your child's symptoms are usually worse after sleeping, mites should be considered.

How to Get Rid of Dust Mites

One of the best ways to reduce dust-mite exposure is to use hypoallergenic mattress and pillow covers. This is a simple, inexpensive, and effective technique. A recent study in *The Journal of Allergy and Clinical Immunology* found that these covers trap allergens while still allowing air to flow through them, which helps absorb perspiration. Covers are also beneficial when your child is allergic to other allergens found in mattresses, such as feathers, cotton, or wool. Covers may even reduce eczema, since dust mites are linked to eczema.

The first generation of mattress and pillow covers were made of uncomfortable plastic. Now, however, several companies have come out with covers made of a tightly woven synthetic fabric. It's not exactly as soft as cotton, but it's pretty close.

Another way to reduce mites is to wash all sheets, blankets, and comforter covers regularly in hot water, which kills dust mites. Weather permitting, area rugs can be brought outside and exposed to the direct sun for an hour or so, which will also kill mites and their eggs.

Researchers have found that using a dehumidifier helps to keep dust-mite levels low. Several studies have shown that mites are unable to survive in environments with 50 percent humidity or less. They are also not well adapted to high altitudes and are not found at levels over 5,000 feet.

Finally, you can remove wall-to-wall carpeting. Carpeting is a major source of dust mites (as well as formaldehyde and mold, as you will read below). Asthmatics do much better if there is no wall-to-wall carpeting anywhere in the house. Sometimes just removing carpeting from a child's bedroom can make an enormous difference. Or, if you don't want to remove any carpeting at all, you can get one of several different types of acaricide (dust-mite-killing) powders or sprays that contain tannic acid. While your child is out of the house, sprinkle the powder on the carpet, let it sit there for a couple of hours, and then vacuum. It's a good idea to wear a mask while you're doing this, as the acidic powder could irritate your respiratory system.

Dust

Dust itself is another major cause of allergies. *Dust* is really just a word to describe airborne particles of fabric, pet dander, insects, dirt, flakes of skin, and other debris. Your child could be allergic to just one component of the dust, such as mouse dander.

How to Get Rid of Dust

The obvious first step is to keep your house clean. Regularly vacuum and dust the house with a damp or oiled cloth, even areas that are normally closed off, such as the basement and attic. Keep your child out of unused rooms that accumulate dust, and keep her out of the house when vacuuming and dusting. If this doesn't help, you may want to invest in a better vacuum cleaner. Vacuums operate by sucking most of the dirt into the bag and blowing used air out the back. Often that exhaust air contains the very things that affect asthmatics the most—tiny particles, including mites and dust. Both Miele and Nilfisk make HEPA vacuum cleaners based on technology used by NASA scientists to ensure that an environment is as dust-free as possible. Electrostatic mops can also pick up the residual dust that vacuums leave behind.

The next step is to have your heating or air-conditioning ducts professionally cleaned regularly to make sure dust doesn't just keeping getting recirculated. Apartment dwellers should be sure to change filters on air-conditioning and heating units regularly.

Consider replacing all your child's stuffed toys with toys that can be washed in a hot washing machine to get rid of dust and dust mites. Or you can keep these toys out of your child's bedroom.

Use air purifiers with HEPA filters (see "The Best Air Filters for Your Home" on page 40) either on the windows or throughout the house. If you live in the city, keep windows closed during peak pollution hours, usually late afternoon. In the country, you might want to keep windows closed during allergy season.

If you plan to renovate your house, make sure you talk to the contractor about controlling the dust and keeping areas being renovated sealed off from the rest of the house.

Mold

Many asthma patients are sensitive to mold spores. Mold produces common allergy symptoms, such as watery eyes and sinus congestion, and can also lead to acute asthma attacks. Molds tend to grow in warm, moist environments, such as beach houses, sand, and in pools of water from common household leaks. A particularly dangerous type of mold called *stachybotrys,* which can cause serious life-threatening illnesses in asthmatics and others, leaves telltale black stains on bathroom and basement walls. In certain buildings in cities, mold is believed to be one of the contributors to *sick building syndrome.* Outdoors, mold increases in the fall from decomposing leaves and after frost in the spring.

If you suspect that mold is a problem in your home, the first step is to buy mold culture plates to determine if toxic levels are present. These are placed in suspect areas of the home, such as the cellar or bathroom, for fifteen to twenty minutes or so, then sent to a lab for a report.

How to Get Rid of Mold
Try to keep the humidity in your home below 50 percent, which is too dry for mold to grow. Ensure that your home has proper drainage, that your foundation and cellar are properly sealed, that gutters are regularly cleaned, and that water isn't leaking from any sinks or bathtub faucets and drains. Keep your bathrooms aired out and dry, even wiping down the walls of the shower after each use. During the summer months, keep

your air conditioners on. Otherwise water will collect in the unit and become a source for mold. Clean evaporation trays and drains in dehumidifiers, air conditioners, furnaces, freezers, and refrigerators. Make sure seals on the doors of the refrigerator are firm to prevent leakage. Ventilate attics, basements, and crawl spaces.

If you use a cold humidifier, be sure to clean it thoroughly, as it can also grow mold and spew the spores into the air. I've seen whole families that have gotten sick from these humidifiers, which are either separate units or attached to central heating systems.

Finally, you might want to consider moving your child's bedroom. A bedroom located on a side of the house where the sun rarely shines will put your child at greater risk. Sun is the perfect antidote to mold growth, and just this change could make all the difference.

Pollen

If your child's asthma comes and goes with the seasons—especially spring and fall—pollen is a likely cause. Pollen has long been known to be a source of asthma attacks. A few hints that the allergy is pollen related: Symptoms flare up in the morning when the child goes outside, they are worse on clear and windy days, and they improve after first frost and inside air-conditioned rooms.

It's important to get your child tested to know which pollen he is allergic to. This can be done with standard allergy skin or blood tests (for more information on allergy testing, see Chapter 4). Trees typically bloom in early spring, late March to early June. Grass tends to pollinate from May to early July. Ragweed spikes after the first week in August and lasts until the middle of October. Different areas of the country have different possible triggers. Corn, for instance, causes many allergic reactions in Iowa.

How to Avoid Pollen

Windows should be kept shut during pollen season, or window air filters should be installed.

Pets

Sometimes it's obvious that a child is allergic to a pet, particularly if the symptoms increase right after a new pet is brought home, or if symptoms are worse when a child is close to a pet. Other times it's not so obvious. Doctors can confirm a pet allergy with allergy tests. There is still confusion as to what exactly causes a pet allergy. Contrary to many people's belief that they are caused by cat or dog hair, allergies are brought on by exposure to dander, a protein found in cat and dog saliva. After cats groom themselves, for instance, they will rub against your legs, furniture, or drapes, depositing dander on your clothes, skin, and home. Dander is sturdy stuff and can last in a home for up to a year. I once had a patient who got a secondhand couch and discovered that dander from the previous owner's dog was causing her allergies.

You should be aware that a recent study has shown that cat exposure early in life may reduce the risk of asthma by desensitizing allergic toddlers. My experience, however, is that this is not the case.

How to Deal with Pet Allergies

Your doctor can discuss all the options available for getting a pet allergy under control. There are a number of steps to consider before finding a new home for the pet. You can restrict the pet from certain parts of the house—for example, strictly forbidding the pet to enter your child's bedroom. Air purifiers and vacuum cleaners with HEPA filters can remove some of the airborne dander. As dander sticks easily to fabrics, eliminating carpets and low-hanging drapes helps. Get slipcovers that you can wash frequently for all your furniture, or invest in leather furniture. Keep your pets off your furniture. There are pet-cleaning products and sprays that can reduce dander. Washing your pet at least twice a week can help, according to an April 1999 report in *The Journal of Allergy and Clinical Immunology.*

Pests

Several recent studies have indicated that some of the most common household triggers for asthma include droppings and body parts of cockroaches, mice, and other rodents. It is essential to reduce your child's exposure to these common household pests. The best way to prevent this exposure is to keep your house clean. Keep all food tightly packaged in plastic or metal containers. Close up cracks in floors, ceilings, and walls to prevent the pests from entering your home. If you can't get rid of pests on your own, employ an expert to remove them, but make sure everyone is out of the house during the extermination. Always try to use nontoxic treatments rather than pesticides or poisons that your child may come in contact with.

CHEMICALS IN YOUR ENVIRONMENT

Formaldehyde

Chemical exposure has increased at an extraordinary pace. We are now confronted with more and different types of chemicals than at any other time in history. Our bodies are being asked to detoxify an ever-increasing list of hazardous substances. One of the most common is formaldehyde. Even though the EPA claims that formaldehyde is a probable cause of cancer, it is still used in a variety of synthetic materials. When new products are installed or new furniture is purchased, it can take up to a year for toxic levels of formaldehyde vapor to dissipate.

Formaldehyde is in shower curtains, cosmetics, detergents, toiletries, and countless other products. The most concentrated source of formaldehyde, however, is found in building materials, furniture, paints, glues, and wallpaper. In sum, your entire home could be completely saturated by these chemical-laden products.

While some companies are developing home-monitoring kits, you will probably need a professional to determine exact levels of formaldehyde in your home. Check the resource area at www.drcity.com for more information on finding an expert who can help.

How to Avoid Formaldehyde Exposure

When possible, it is best to avoid using products that are high in formaldehyde in your home in the first place. When doing any renovations in your home, there are nontoxic alternatives. Instead of using oil- or solvent-based paints, for instance, try water-based paints, which are considered less toxic and emit far fewer illness-provoking fumes. Builders are already replacing plywood with waferboard, which releases much less formaldehyde into your home. Using natural paints and avoiding carpeting significantly decreases allergic symptoms.

If you do suspect high levels of formaldehyde, ventilate your house as much as possible. Some authorities recommend using ozone-filter machines, which can neutralize formaldehyde in the air. Ozone, however, can be irritating to the lungs, and these devices should not be left on while an asthmatic is in the room.

Carbon Monoxide

This invisible gas is a by-product of combustion. It can leak into your home through chimneys, fireplaces, woodstoves, or inadequately sealed heating systems. Carbon monoxide interferes with oxygen delivery to the body, and as asthmatics already have trouble breathing, this can exacerbate it. Carbon monoxide produces flulike symptoms, as well as headaches, dizziness, and increased heart rate. Inexpensive carbon-monoxide detectors are available at most hardware stores and are now considered as essential as fire detectors. Certain air filters come with built-in carbon-monoxide detectors for your house.

How to Avoid Carbon-Monoxide Exposure

Check fireplace flues frequently to be sure they are clean and unblocked, and keep garage doors sealed from the rest of the house. If you live in an apartment dwelling, be aware that air conditioners can draw in exhaust from nearby traffic or parking garages. Good ventilation is key here.

Cleaning Products

Vapors from common cleaners can cause throat and lung irritation along with burning of the eyes, nose, and throat in healthy adults. For asthmatic children, this only pours salt in the wound. Most of these cleaners, disinfectants, and air fresheners contain chemicals like ammonia, ethanol, or acetone. These toxic chemicals can sensitize an asthmatic child's lungs, because they are often delivered through aerosolized mists that can be drawn deeply into the lungs, causing serious irritation and damage. This is another reason to keep your child out of the house when cleaning is taking place, and why it's important to keep cleaning supplies well out of the reach of children and to keep your supplies tightly capped and closed. There are mild cleansers that are much less toxic, such as

Simple Green and Envirocide, which are available in health food stores and grocery stores. Using these will benefit everyone, including your asthmatic child.

Chlorine found in bleach can cause significant irritation to the nose, throat, and lungs. When combined with decaying matter, chlorine can produce a compound called *chloroform,* which is a carcinogen. Immediately reduce the use of chlorinated products, and to further reduce your child's exposure, install a filter on your main water supply line or at the tap for drinking water.

Ammonia is another major irritant used in cleaning. Check bottle labels for ammonia content. Exposure causes irritation of the eyes, nose, throat, and respiratory tract; eye and skin burns; and chest pains. Always use it in a well-ventilated area. If you or your child comes in contact with ammonia, immediately wash the skin with soap and water. Never mix ammonia and chlorine, as they can cause toxic fumes when combined.

Ozone

There is a lot of confusion about ozone. In the upper atmosphere, ozone provides a protective layer to filter out ultraviolet radiation from the sun. Without that layer, the earth would simply burn up. Closer to the earth, however, greenhouse gases combine with sunlight and oxygen to create ozone. This street-level ozone is a health hazard. Low levels of ozone can produce coughing; moderate levels can trigger chest pain, nasal congestion, and shortness of breath. Asthmatics are known to be especially sensitive to ozone. Countless electrical machines, such as photocopiers, produce it. If your home has many of these machines—say, for a home office—keep them all in one well-ventilated room.

Asbestos

While most asbestos has been banned in certain building materials for a number of years, there are many older homes that contain asbestos insulation in electrical systems, walls, and even in tiles. In most cases, asbestos won't cause any problems; however, if you do have asbestos in your home, be sure to seal it off as securely as possible. It's when you disturb asbestos that the fibers get into the air and the lungs. If removal is contemplated, a certified asbestos-removal company should do it. Call the EPA asbestos hotline at 1–800–368–5888.

How to Detoxify Your Child's School

A sick school can negate much of the work you do at home to eliminate toxins. But few schools are willing to overhaul their entire building for the sake of an asthmatic child. In a perfect world, you could ask your school to use nontoxic alternatives to cleaning chemicals. Mice and cockroach problems would be eliminated, and a pest-prevention program would be put in place. Schools with inadequate ventilation or poor water quality would be cleaned up. Your child's classroom would be free from chalk or other dust and odors from glues and paints. When renovations are done, schools would use nontoxic products whenever possible, and the area would be sealed off and ventilated. While it's unlikely that you'll be able to convince your school administrator to do all of this, you may win a few battles. To protect your child, you'll need to take a proactive stance at school and keep complaining until you get a response. Asthmatic children have a right to an environment that is safe and doesn't make them sick.

THE BEST AIR FILTERS FOR YOUR HOME

An important defense against sick air is a top-quality air filter. Fortunately, a new generation of air-filtering and -purifying systems is now available that can reduce everything from toxic vapors to dust to tiny particles of soot. Many of these new filters are also much quieter and more efficient than their predecessors.

The most common type of portable air filter contains a HEPA filter. HEPA filters, originally used only in operating rooms, trap pollen and dust as small as 0.01 microns. Theoretically, they remove 90 percent of all dust and pollen in the air. HEPA filters are the only ones to eliminate dust-mite particles and have been shown in several studies to reduce allergic respiratory symptoms. More powerful appliances made by Austin Air and Honeywell (Enviracaire) have a charcoal filter in addition to a HEPA filter. A charcoal filter can not only capture some larger particles but will also neutralize chemicals such as benzene, chlorine, and formaldehyde.

There are window filters that can filter air from outside and are particularly useful in spring and fall, when there is a lot of pollen circulating outside. Air-conditioning units will also remove a great deal of pollen and dust. In humid climates, condensation that builds up in the unit could cause mold to grow. In this case, you should keep the fan on at all times.

Keep in mind that asthmatics in winter climates may need a humidifier during the cold part of the year. Keeping humidity at the proper level is important for asthmatics, as ultra-dry air can provoke an asthma attack and very humid air can promote dust mites and mold growth.

It's a good idea to install an electrostatic filter in your furnace to filter the air in your entire house. These filters should be changed once or twice a year, or washed every month with a hose. If you have forced-air heat or central air-conditioning, you can put electrostatic filters on vents, which, if you replace them every couple of months, will cut down on dust significantly.

Where to Get Allergy Products and Air Filters

For more information on where to obtain environmental testing and allergy control products, visit the Asthma and Allergy Resources Section and the Health Store at www.drcity.com.

chapter four

Food—The Good, the Bad, and the Ugly

What your child eats can have a profound effect on her asthma. For one thing, she could have a food allergy that is making the illness worse. Second, a good diet is crucial to the overall health of growing children. Third, eating certain nutritious foods appears to have a positive effect on asthmatic symptoms in children. Finally, some foods can provoke gastroesophageal reflux, which can trigger an attack. While many doctors scoff at the benefits of good nutrition for asthmatics, I wouldn't be surprised if someday soon many of the same dietary guidelines that are now in place for cancer and heart disease are extended to asthma.

I know that putting an asthma-fighting meal plan in place isn't easy. Kids are picky eaters and certainly won't switch to a diet rich in fruits and vegetables in a day. You need to dissect and study your child's food patterns to isolate the culprits. When I start discussing nutrition with parents, they often sit there with their eyes wide open and think, "Oh my God, we had no idea so many factors are involved."

Relax. It's important to take this as a step-by-step process. Below I lay out the nutritional part of my Breath of Life program that parents have been successfully following for years. It will help you employ nutrition as a high-tech medicine to give your child's body precisely what it needs at a cellular level to protect and heal itself. It will educate you about the major causes of allergy or sensitivity in children and help you to methodically unearth any food-related allergies in your child. Yes, my dietary recommendations require some diligence, but from my observations over the years, I believe you ignore nutrition at your child's peril. (For more information on getting your family to eat well and other health issues, visit the Message Board at: www.drcity.com.)

Last year I treated a seven-year-old boy named Oliver who'd had asthma for a while. He just kept getting sick with frequent colds and wheezing and even had made a few recent trips to the emergency room. There didn't appear to be any pattern to his sickness, so it didn't seem to be attributable to an allergen like peanuts or pollen. As I took a background history of Oliver and interviewed his parents, I discovered that he had a terrible diet. The family ate fast-food dinners regularly, snacks consisted of soda and cookies, and breakfast was often some sugary treat like doughnuts or Danishes. Almost everything the family ate came out of a box.

Oliver's parents were reluctant to make too many changes at once and preferred to follow the Breath of Life program one step at a time. Slowly his parents were able to get him to eat healthy foods such as salads, raw vegetables, whole-grain breads, fruits, and fish. It took some coaxing and experimentation to find foods he would eat, but with the help of my nutritional counselor, Oliver was eating a much better diet in a few weeks' time. The change was dramatic: His frequent cold symptoms were eliminated, and he soon even felt good enough to join Little League. His parents have started to introduce other parts of the Breath of Life program, and now, more than a year later, Oliver hasn't had any exacerbation of his asthma, and he continues to improve and excel.

✢ Does Your Child Have Gastroesophageal Reflux? ✢

As in adults, reflux esophagitis can be a hidden reason for asthma. Symptoms in children include stomachaches, frequent coughing, spontaneous stomachaches in the evening or morning, and shortness of breath during the night.

Reflux occurs when stomach acids flow back through a small valve that opens into the esophagus. A bacterium, *H. pylori*, which has been implicated in stomach ulcers, has also been evident in patients with reflux. The cells of our stomachs are designed to withstand exposure to this powerful hydrochloric acid. This is not true for the delicate cells lining the esophagus or the upper airways. Once acid backwashes into the esophagus, it can seep into the throat. From there, it can cause direct damage to the lungs, ultimately injuring the delicate tissue found in the lungs. Reflux can also severely irritate the nasal passages, pharynx, and vocal cords, as well as cause chronic sore throats.

The process of elimination usually diagnoses reflux. I saw five-year-old Kyle from upstate New York recently, and no one could figure out why he had suffered a relapse. One morning, with his usual milk and Cheerios, Kyle suffered an attack. We tested him for milk allergy, but it was negative. When he had another flare-up, we noticed that it happened at the same time of day. This time Kyle also complained of a stomachache. As we knew he wasn't allergic to milk, we realized that the most likely culprit was reflux. After we discontinued regular milk and substituted rice-based milk, Kyle's symptoms went away. By keeping a diary and understanding the many factors that cause asthma, we were able to solve the problem.

Symptoms from reflux usually occur after meals, but often the acid can flow back while your child is sleeping or lying down. There are certain foods that tend to increase reflux in adults—including citrus, peppermint, tomatoes, caffeine, chocolate, and certain spices—but children may have reflux for additional reasons. Lactose-intolerant children suffer from excess gas when they drink milk, and this can predispose them to reflux. Eating just before sleeping can also increase the risk of reflux.

The Best Diet for Asthmatics

When was the last time you heard the words *nutrition* and *asthma* in the same sentence? Probably never. Many physicians still think diet has no effect on asthma. Nothing could be further from the truth. Just last summer, a study from Saudi Arabia made headlines because researchers discovered that junk-food-eating city kids had a higher risk of asthma than children from rural areas, where the diet still consists of rice, lamb, and fresh produce. Those children who had the lowest intakes of vegetables, milk, vitamin E, and certain minerals, the study found, were at significantly greater risk of asthma, even after adjusting for other factors. "This study suggests that dietary factors during childhood are an important influence in determining the expression of wheezy illness," the authors concluded. While more research is needed, there are now an increasing number of physicians who believe nutrition can have a significant impact on the health and longevity of asthmatics.

Yet bad nutrition is rarely mentioned as a contributing factor to asthma. One reason may be that asthma is poorly understood. It's reasonably easy to grasp the idea that calcium builds bones, that fat clogs arteries, and that certain vitamins—including E and C—may prevent cancer. Unlike a clogged artery, however, asthma is not a simple mechanical problem. The link between diet and asthma is now becoming clearer as more and more research comes to light.

After my nearly fatal asthma attack, I eliminated every single food I thought was harming me. I knew my body needed as much help as possible, and I tried to flood my system with healthy nutrients. I took extreme care to avoid food I was allergic to. I stopped eating processed and junk foods. I ate mostly fish, fresh produce, whole grains, and free-range chicken. Now, years later, I can look back at my asthmatic crisis and see that it was a blessing in disguise, one that forced me to see the importance of nutrition.

I've spent much of my professional life studying nutritional medicine so that I could learn about the power of different foods and share this knowledge with my patients. My book *The Nutraceutical Revolution* (Riverhead, 1999) explains in detail how specific nutrients have the capacity to act like medicines. In many ways, they are *natural* pharmaceuticals. In the book, I talk about the recent scientific advances that have unlocked the mysteries of healing foods and nutrients, giving us the tools to make full use of nature's medicine chest. Researchers now study and isolate the chemical composition of fruits, berries, vegetables, herbs, fish, and poultry. We are beginning to understand how nutrients affect our cells, our organs, our blood, even our DNA—and how they protect us from disease.

We seem to be bombarded with reports on the everyday miracles of nutrition. Soybeans lower cholesterol. Tomatoes cut the risk of prostate cancer. Folic acid prevents *spina bifida*. Fish oil slows the growth of colon tumors. We have learned that within hours after eating broccoli, sulforaphane courses through the bloodstream, activating enzymes that literally whisk carcinogens out of the cells so the body can discard them.

Some research has targeted asthma. In April 2000, *Thorax* reported that eating vitamin-rich fruits like oranges "may reduce wheezing symptoms in childhood, especially among already susceptible individuals." A recent study found that the risk of bronchial irritation was increased sevenfold among those with the lowest intake of vitamin C in their diets. People in the study who ate the least saturated fats, on the other hand, had a much lower chance of suffering from asthma. There are conflicting data on other foods, such as fish oil, but from my experience it is clear that patients who eat well get better.

The sorry truth is that most children eat too much junk food. For many kids, the only source of vitamins is breakfast cereals that have been fortified with vitamins, which is sadly still probably better than what they are offered at school. Since the 1980s, there has been a rapidly growing trend to target children as consumers. As a result, in 2001 children in the United States spent nearly $10 billion of their own money on food and beverages (junk food), and their parents were persuaded to spend close to $110 billion. So great is this problem worldwide, that it is now receiving attention from the World Health Organization—the issue: How can we encourage kids (and their parents) to redirect that spending to healthier foods and goods?

Junk food is especially bad for asthmatic children. You probably already know that junk and many processed foods contain refined sugar and fats, such as trans-saturated fats and saturated fats. Junk food, as you know, can make your child listless or hyperactive and contribute to a host of other health problems. But evidence suggests that the fats mentioned above may promote the formation of harmful prostaglandins, which cause inflammation. Junk food can also lead to excess weight, which has been found to contribute to asthma. One recent study found that weight loss in obese patients reduced airway obstruction in those with asthma.

Kids are not programmed to eat Froot Loops instead of apples. While most kids appreciate a treat now and then, it's not something they inherently crave or demand constantly. I've always been surprised to see how easily the children I work with adapt to a healthy diet. Sometimes parents have a harder time with this diet revolution than do their children.

If children are taught early on that carrots, grapes, raisins, and nuts (if they're not allergic) are treats, you'll go a long way toward getting them into the habit of good nutrition. Remember that you're in control here. If you don't buy Oreos, there are no Oreos to eat. Because you determine what goes in the refrigerator, you can control their diets for at least the first five or six years of their life. Sure, it's hard to avoid junk food at parties and on holidays, but if the focus at home is on good-tasting, nutritious food, the junk food will be reduced to an occasional thing.

One way to make it easier is to get across the idea that this is a partnership between you and your child, that you are both working toward the same goal, and that you are doing this together for everyone's benefit. Explain to your child why certain foods can make asthma (and related allergies) better or worse. Talk to your kids about what they should eat: whole grains, not white bread or white-flour cakes. Fresh and steamed vegetables. Fresh fruit, not canned fruit and juices, which contain sugar and other additives. Poultry, fish, lean beef hamburgers, and healthy vegetable oils. Not only can these foods improve your child's overall health, but compounds within many foods can help cut down on free radicals, powerful molecules that can damage your child's lungs and immune system (see "What Are Free Radicals?" on page 88). In Chapter 6, you'll read about the mounting body of evidence that indicates how specific substances in foods can greatly improve an asthmatic's health.

Work with your child to eliminate foods that are potentially the most problematic, including cookies and candies. Explain how some foods make most people feel yucky, tired, hyper, or congested. Ask your child if she can think of any food that makes her feel like this. Explain why foods that are fatty, greasy, and sugary are not good for them. Fatty fried foods, for instance, are toxic for everyone because they clog our arteries and promote free-radical damage. Describe how fatty food contributes to excess weight and lowers our energy level. Tell your child that these foods are especially bad for her because they may promote inflammatory reactions in the lungs. It's pretty easy for kids to understand that french fries are drenched in bad oils and have very little nutritional benefit at all. You don't have to hit kids over the head with the idea that eating better equals feeling better.

For example, take the kids I worked with in the school in the Bronx. These kids were used to eating junk food, yet they quickly became savvy about their diets and soon understood that eating wasn't just about taste but also about health. While we didn't monitor their food consumption outside of school, they all became much more aware of what was good for them and what wasn't. They became agents of change for their families, encouraging their parents to buy better foods. They knew that this was an important part of the program and accepted it as part of the process. On the very last day of the program, we had a graduation ceremony at which we served only healthy foods—fruit, yogurt dip, and vegetables like broccoli and carrots. Every bite was gone at the end of the day. That's what was there; that's what they ate.

Finally, never lose sight of the fact that children are growing and need lots of food, especially high-energy foods such as pasta, rice, and potatoes. While you want to carefully monitor what your children eat, you should focus on getting as much quality food as you can into their systems and ensuring that they maintain a positive attitude about meals and eating.

IDENTIFYING FOOD ALLERGIES

Asthmatic children account for a disproportionate share of the estimated 3 to 8 percent of all children who have food allergies. More kids have allergies than adults, possibly because their immature digestive tracts may not be able to process food properly. Food allergies are a nasty and often unsuspected culprit for many childhood illnesses. A 1994 study from Georgetown University, for example, found that nearly 80 percent of chronic ear infections could be linked to food allergies. Infections are an important concern for asthmatic children, whether they be ear infections or lung infections.

Certain foods are more likely to cause allergic reactions than others. While it's possible that your child could be allergic to almost anything, the most common foods that cause a reaction, according to the National Institutes of Health, include eggs, milk, and peanuts. I also have many patients who are allergic to corn, soy, chocolate, and wheat. Other people may be allergic to shellfish or certain fruits. Indeed, the possibilities are endless.

The difficulty with identifying food allergies is that so much of the American diet is processed food, which can contain any number of hidden ingredients. Consider a child with a corn allergy. His parents may studiously avoid every food that contains corn, only to find that corn syrup was hidden in their favorite can of peaches. Or it is in the cookies and candies their kids regularly snack on. If you have a child with a food allergy, this means you have to carefully read every single nutrition label on every package of food that enters the house. Fortunately, most children with asthma are not this allergic to food.

Not every food comes with a label, however. Bagels and fresh breads, food at bake sales, food at restaurants, and meals at friends' houses are all potential time bombs. Many breads use soy flour or may contain dairy or corn products. I once treated a child who visited a friend whose mother knew about the child's allergy to milk. Yet she absentmindedly served fish fried in a prepackaged batter that contained some dried milk powder. When the child became ill, everyone was perplexed until they went through every item the child ate.

Foods can also be inadvertently contaminated with other foods in the manufacturing process. Cross-contamination can occur anywhere from the delivery truck to the factory. A lot of chocolate candy, for instance, contains traces of peanut. Chocolate bars are made in the same vats as chocolate and peanut bars, so even after the vats are cleaned, there is no way to make sure the entire assembly line of machines and tools has been cleaned of all peanut residue. As a result, most chocolate products are now labeled "May contain traces of peanut." Parents should take this warning seriously.

In addition to allergies, there are substances in foods that your child may be sensitive to, including MSG, sulfites, and yellow dye #5 (tartrazine). Sensitivities and allergies often present confusingly similar symptoms, but both can provoke a severe asthmatic response. Allergies are usually easier to detect, because they tend to produce more obvious symptoms and cause your body to produce immunoglobulin-E (IgE) antibodies that can be detected through a blood or skin test. Sensitivities are much more difficult to isolate, since they do not produce a measurable antibody reaction. Your doctor can help you identify which is which, either through blood tests or through the process of elimination. Keeping a diary of your child's symptoms is also very helpful.

The causes for allergies are not well understood. Some experts suspect that exposure to certain foods within the first year of life can promote later allergic reactions. Others claim that certain allergies can be traced back to what a child's mother ate during pregnancy; preliminary evidence suggests that the diets of some pregnant women cause their children to be predisposed to allergies. Other factors include the allergic histories of both parents.

Food allergies can be serious and occasionally even life-threatening. Certain children with peanut allergies, for example, can go into anaphylactic shock, which is characterized by swelling in the throat and respiratory tract and a drop in blood pressure. Many schools, in fact, have banned peanut butter because of the high risk of anaphylaxis. As many as one in 100 young children are allergic to peanuts, and most schools are simply not willing to take on the risk that a student could have an anaphylactic reaction because he takes a bite of another kid's sandwich.

How do you know if your child suffers from food allergies? Symptoms usually include recurrent headaches, skin rashes, fatigue or irritability, itching after eating, wheezing, or shortness of breath. Some allergies are obvious—a skin rash every time your child eats strawberries, for instance—and some are harder to pinpoint, such as frequent ear infections in a child with corn allergies.

If you think food allergies are a problem, allergy tests are a worthwhile first step. Your doctor can administer a painless prick or skin test, which I find extremely helpful. An extract of the offending food is injected or scratched under the skin to see if the child develops a welt in response. The size of the welt is then compared with a control and evaluated by your doctor to see if it is within normal range.

Some doctors suggest certain blood tests called radioallergosorbent test (RAST). These tests may be safer than skin tests for children who are experiencing asthmatic symptoms. They are especially suitable for children who've had any serious reactions to foods, who have persistent skin rashes that might obscure results, or who have a risk of an acute asthmatic attack during testing. RAST measures allergic potential by determining the total amount of IgE in your child's blood. IgE are antibodies that often develop after repeated exposure to a particular food or allergen. Theoretically, the higher the IgE level in the child's blood, the more allergic he is. This can help to isolate the offending substance. Some doctors recommend both tests, since they may detect different al-

lergens. These same blood and skin tests are also used to identify environmental allergies.

But food allergy tests aren't perfect, particularly with children.
Younger children's immune systems are still developing, and even though
a child may have an allergic reaction to a particular substance, she could
still have a negative blood or skin test. I've tested children who have a
history of shortness of breath after eating peanuts who still test negative
on the scratch tests or RAST. Frequently these tests may turn positive
later in life. As they're not infallible, it's best to consider allergy tests as
an additional diagnostic tool rather than the final word.

You may want to manipulate your child's diet to try to isolate offending foods. Obviously, if you know your child is allergic to milk or peanuts,
you should avoid those foods. But when it's difficult to pinpoint the ori-
gin of more subtle reactions, a special diet can help. I usually just suggest a diet that eliminates any possible suspects for a week or two, and
then gradually rotates them back in, one by one, to see if anything
causes a reaction. Or if you think your child is allergic to many foods,
you might want to isolate one or two major areas. For example, you
might avoid soy, wheat, and milk but keep on eating corn and eggs. A lot
depends on your child's ability to comply. Sometimes, reducing something 50 percent can lessen a child's symptoms significantly; other times
total elimination is required. While you're doing this, it's important to
keep a journal noting what your child eats at each meal, when symptoms
start, and what the specific reactions are. Over time, patterns will emerge
that will shorten your search for the allergy-causing culprits.

When an allergy is identified, many parents have trouble figuring out
what to substitute for such common foods as wheat or milk. You'll find
plenty of choices at your local health food store and, increasingly, at regular supermarkets. Instead of wheat, for example, you can substitute
spelt and quinoa cereals, pastas, and breads. Many children find these
quite delicious. Your child can drink soy instead of milk, or rice-based

milk instead of soy. Don't become discouraged if the product is not up to your kid's standards. Try a new brand or product, and keep trying until you find something your kid likes. There are plenty of manufacturers out there trying to corner the growing market of people with food allergies, and you might be surprised at the wide selection of *healthy* foods that actually taste good.

❧ Five Ways to Get Your Kids to Eat Right ❧

1. Keep a chart in the kitchen of foods that are good for growing bodies and that your child enjoys. This will help him visualize the connection between health and a good diet.

2. Put healthy and nonhealthy foods on a paper towel overnight to see which ones soak the towel with fatty grease. Suggestions include a carrot, a french fry, a Ritz cracker, popcorn with butter, and popcorn without. This illustrates how much more fats some foods have than others and lets your kids see the fat in living color.

3. Have your child draw pictures of healthful foods to hang on the walls of the kitchen. For example, she can draw a picture of a tomato, corn, or a fruit basket.

4. Take a trip to the health food store and get your child involved in the weekly shopping. Work out a daily menu of foods that make him feel great.

5. Put a plate of cut vegetables on the table fifteen minutes before each meal is served. When there's nothing else to eat and the kids are hungry, they'll eat the carrots, celery, red pepper strips, and cucumber wheels.

chapter five

Asthma Medication and Kids

Medicating children is a tricky business. There is no question that in acute situations, drugs are lifesavers. For many asthmatics, they provide a bridge to a healthier life. On the other hand, we don't know enough about the long-term effects of many potent asthma medicines on growing bodies. The Breath of Life program provides a natural approach to coping with asthma, but it is important for parents to have a general overview of the more common asthma medications. Every time your child is prescribed an asthma drug, you need to weigh the risk of the drug's long-term side effects against the risk of this serious illness.

All too often, however, parents aren't informed about the drugs their kids are taking. For instance, inhaled steroids are one of the most common classes of medications for asthmatics. Many parents of asthmatic children were no doubt happy to read an October 2000 report in *Time* magazine that proclaimed, "Inhaled steroids now seem to be safe for children with moderate asthma." Inhaled steroids (or *corticosteroids,* as they are known in the scientific community) are perhaps the best option we have for people who need to get moderate to severe symptoms under control. Indeed, I often prescribe them for short-term use, and inhaled steroids do have a place in the long-term treatment of asthma for certain patients. *Time* noted the promising results of two recent studies in *The New England Journal of Medicine (NEJM)* suggesting that steroids don't cause long-term growth suppression. Even though steroid-inhaling kids may stop growing for a while, they eventually catch up.

Time didn't tell the whole story, however. While the studies do hold out the hope that inhaled steroids are safe for short-term use, an editorial in the same issue of *NEJM* noted that the researchers hadn't discovered *why* these drugs hindered growth temporarily, nor did they evaluate the drug's long-term effects on other organs, such as the brain, liver, and lungs. The number of *alveoli,* or air sacs in the lung, increases by a factor of six after birth and keeps multiplying until sometime between age five and eight. Ingesting steroids during this crucial time may actually decrease lung cell mass. The *NEJM* editorial concluded that due to "the sparseness of data on the influence of corticosteroids on organ development . . . it may be prudent to avoid the use of inhaled corticosteroids in young children with very mild asthma."

This is in sharp contrast to optimistic media reports. Why is this so? Well, we all like a quick fix. Many parents, once they see how well asthma medications initially appear to work, lose their incentive to eliminate every possible asthma trigger in the house and keep up with the breathing lessons. Medications appear to be the easy route.

Now, don't get me wrong. Drugs are not the bad guys. I am the first person to tell you that asthma needs to be treated aggressively when it seriously endangers health. Often medical intervention is necessary to put a child back on track. If a child is frequently having asthmatic episodes and they're disrupting her life, an inhaled steroid may be worthwhile. Other asthma medications, such as bronchodilators and leukotriene inhibitors, are also useful. Certainly, if your child is still sick after assiduously following my asthma program, you could argue that the risk of *not* using medications is too high. In no case should you reduce or eliminate your child's medication without discussing it thoroughly with your child's physician.

The problem is that too often asthma medications—both steroids and others—are prescribed without any plan for reducing or eliminating them once your child is on them. As a result, parents of asthmatic kids feel trapped. They think they are left with the choice of unknown side effects of drugs, on one hand, and the risk of asthma attacks on the other. This is simply not true.

I believe parents have other choices. While you should never change your child's drug regimen without consulting your doctor, it may be possible to wean your child off drugs for good. If you become educated about the risks and benefits of asthma drugs, you can create a plan that will help you rely on them when necessary and at the same time seek ways to reduce the need for drugs.

You also need to remember that one year's miracle treatment may be the next year's discarded therapy. In the 1980s, for instance, theophylline was considered the drug of choice for asthma, mainly because it is effective and cheap. Theophylline needs to be carefully monitored through regular blood tests, however, which makes it a difficult drug to administer to children. I remember seeing a ten-year-old child named Julia, whose mother, Barbara, noted that she was irritable and constantly suffering from nausea. When I asked about medications, Barbara explained that Julia was on a slow-release theophylline preparation. During the exam, Julia seemed anxious, unfocused, and distracted whenever I asked her a question. Barbara explained that Julia never used to be like this, and she attributed this personality change to the asthma. Barbara also admitted that she kept putting off the required blood tests because Julia reacted violently to needles.

I suspected that Julia's problems were probably due to the theophylline, which many doctors were beginning to suspect was more trouble than it was worth. I immediately discontinued the medication and started Julia on a different therapy. At the same time, after much cajoling, Julia finally agreed to a blood test. Sure enough, her theophylline levels were in the toxic range, which is why she was so nauseous and cranky. Within days of going off theophylline, Julia's symptoms subsided dramatically. Then, with the help of her family, I put Julia on the Breath of Life program, and she continued to get better. In the end, Barbara just needed to be guided through the maze of asthma medications. By learning more about the side effects of the drug her daughter was taking, she was able to make much better choices for her child.

The goal of my Breath of Life program is to help my patients feel well and then to help them reduce or eliminate medications, if possible. Until your child reaches this point, however, the following information will help you to know why your doctor recommends a certain drug, how it works, and its most common side effects. With this information, you will then be able to monitor your child's medicines with wisdom and confidence.

THE MOST COMMON ASTHMA DRUGS FOR KIDS

While this book deals primarily with natural approaches, a discussion of asthma medication is crucial. In general, asthma medications fall into two categories: *anti-inflammatory drugs* and *bronchodilators*. While there are new drugs coming on the market, they generally fall into these two categories. Anti-inflammatory medications (including steroids and nonsteroidal anti-inflammatories such as leukotriene inhibitors and cromolyn sodium) are used to reduce or prevent underlying inflammation but will not immediately open airways. There are believed to be two distinct phases of the *inflammatory cascade,* an early and a late phase. The early phase can begin anywhere from two to twenty-four hours after an attack; the late phase can occur as late as two weeks after an event. Both oral and inhaled steroids are prescribed for both the early and the late phase; cromolyn sodium works on the late phase, and leukotriene inhibitors are designed just for the early phase. Bronchodilators (beta-agonists such as albuterol and salmeterol) are prescribed to open up airways but do not reduce inflammation.

Parents should assume that every asthma drug has side effects, and any abnormal behaviors or symptoms should immediately be reported to your physician.

STEROIDS

When Your Doctor May Prescribe Steroids

Steroids are for patients with chronic or severe asthma. The drug can be taken in three different forms: *intravenously,* via an *inhaled spray,* or *orally* (pills). Intravenous steroids are reserved primarily for the emergency room.

Inhaled steroid sprays are the most common steroid drugs prescribed. These sprays, which have many fewer side effects and potential long-term complications than oral or intravenous steroids, are recommended to prevent symptoms and reduce inflammation in patients with chronic asthma and are not recommended for emergencies. They are considered safer because they are designed to target the lungs only, whereas oral and intravenous steroids are absorbed throughout the body. Inhaled steroids come in a wide variety of brands and dosages. The most common steroid sprays include *beclomethasone* (Beclovent, Vanceril), as well as newer sprays such as *fluticasone* (Flovent), *budesonide* (Pulmicort), *flunisolide* (Aerobid), *triamcinolone* (Azmacort) and newer combination therapies such as Advair (*fluticasone* and *salmeterol*).

Patients may need to try several different brands until they find the one that works best. We are still learning which sprays work best for children and which have the least side effects. Since most have been tested on adults only, dosing children is something of a guessing game in which we try to get the most results with the fewest side effects. One study of twenty-three children found that beclomethasone was more effective than fluticasone but fluticasone was safer than beclomethasone. Some studies indicate that budesonide has less chance of suppressing growth than does beclomethasone.

Oral steroids (pills) should be prescribed for much shorter periods of time than inhaled steroids. They are prescribed after an acute attack, when ongoing symptoms have not been resolved by other means, or when certain tests indicate trouble, such as a 50 percent drop in peak-flow meter readings in a twenty-four-hour period. There are two types of oral steroids that are prescribed for children, *methylprednisolone* and *prednisone*. These drugs are very similar in terms of their effectiveness, though physicians may vary in their prescribing habits. Generally these medications should be prescribed for several weeks, at most, after an acute attack. Aggressive use of steroids at an early stage of an asthma attack can prevent further injury and reduce the likelihood that the condition will worsen.

While there is some disagreement as to what time of day a patient should take oral steroids, most physicians believe they should be taken in the morning, to mimic the body's normal hormonal spike. Other doctors believe the pills should be prescribed in split doses to provide continuous coverage; so a patient would take equal amounts two to four times a day. Another group of physicians believe oral steroids should be taken when symptoms are the most severe, which, for most children, is at night. In this case, a child would take a single dose between four and six in the afternoon to last through the night. I believe all three of these methods may be appropriate, depending on the child and his symptoms.

It is extremely rare for a steroid drug to cause an allergic reaction, but parents should be aware that it occasionally happens. Always contact your physician if you suspect that your child is having an adverse reaction to steroids or any other drug. One question remains about the long-term effectiveness and repeated use of both inhaled and oral steroids: A study of 863 patients at the University of Alberta in Canada reported that prescribing children inhaled or oral steroids within an hour of getting to an emergency room reduced the need for hospitalization. But they found that the people who responded best to the medication had never been on steroids before.

How Steroids Work

When a child is having trouble breathing because of an acute asthma attack, steroids can literally snatch her from the jaws of death. Steroids are synthetic versions of hormones that the body produces naturally, and they work by stopping inflammation. Studies have shown that steroids decrease the production of *cytokines,* an important part of the inflammatory cascade. Steroids have a number of other positive attributes. They can lead to a decreased need for other medications, including the beta-agonist albuterol. Researchers at Montreal Children's Hospital discovered that inhaled steroids enhance lung capacity and improve quality of life more than beta-agonist drugs.

The Most Common Side Effects of Steroids

There is no question that long-term use of oral steroids leads to complications. Medical research indicates that extensive use of oral steroids can irreversibly affect nearly every organ in the body, leading to immune depression, poor wound healing, thinning of the skin, heart and lung damage, weight gain, high blood pressure, thinning of the bones (osteoporosis), joint pain, stomach bleeding, changes in fat metabolism, acne, extra hair growth, stunted growth in children, cataracts, mood disorders, suppression of the adrenal glands, leaching of important minerals like potassium, calcium, and magnesium, and swelling of the face and ankles.

Further, since most studies on oral steroids have been done on adults, we don't have hard-and-fast pediatric dosage guidelines. These medicines are hormones, which can affect children very differently from the way they affect adults, and boys differently from girls. If an adult has an asthma attack, the recommendation is to start him on a fairly high dose of steroids that may equal or surpass the dose limit recommended by the manufacturer. This dose is generally in the 5- to 60-milligram range. The dosage for children between the ages of six and twelve should generally be no higher than 30 milligrams.The belief is that during an acute event, the best thing to do is to treat aggressively to prevent the inflammatory cascade. But while a similar approach may be good for children, the amount and duration of steroid treatment is not well defined. Many of these drugs are not even recommended for children under six years of age.

Inhaled steroids also have side effects. It was originally thought that inhaled steroids selectively targeted the lungs and for that reason were safe. We now know that this isn't entirely true. Inhaled steroids can be absorbed throughout the body as well, which can lead to some of the same problems caused by oral steroids.

Both the *Archives of Internal Medicine* and the *Lancet* recently reported that repeated use of inhaled steroids leads to a decrease in bone mass and puts patients at risk for osteoporosis. The *NEJM* noted that high doses of inhaled cortisone are associated with an increased risk for an invasive pulmonary fungal infection. Researchers found that inhaled steroids promote yeast infections. The journal *Ophthalmology* found that the higher the dose of inhaled steroids, the higher the risk of glaucoma, especially if there is a family history of the eye disease. Cataracts are another risk of prolonged exposure to inhaled steroids. Inhalants can also cause chronic coughing.

Of particular concern to parents and children is the question of growth suppression. Even if the drugs don't affect long-term growth, we know that when children are on inhaled steroids, their growth can be temporarily halted. In an *Annals of Asthma, Allergy and Immunology* study of twenty-six asthmatic children on inhaled steroids, seven showed a decline in growth over the six-month period of the study. A report from Stanford University's Department of Pediatrics found that beclomethasone decreased growth in children during the fifty-four weeks that the study took place.

The bottom line is you need to strike the right balance and work with your doctor to determine when and how steroids should be used for treating asthma in your child. Parents must assess the risks of administering steroids to their children and make an informed decision about their use. In certain situations, there is no better alternative to steroids. In fact, I am sometimes put in the position of urging parents who are afraid of steroids to go ahead and give their children the drugs. Early, aggressive treatment with steroids can often prevent the need for further steroids or other drugs later on, and can also get the patient healthier faster.

At the same time, I consider steroids a short-term, temporary solution. As soon as my patients get over the crisis, I advise them to move on to identifying and removing the triggers for the asthma in the hopes that they won't need steroids again. I also look to substitute other asthma drugs, such as cromolyn sodium, which appear to have fewer side effects. Steroids have an appropriate place in the treatment of asthma, but they should be restricted to the times when the risks involved are worth it.

CROMOLYN SODIUM

When Your Doctor May Prescribe Cromolyn Sodium

Cromolyn sodium is used for children with mild to moderate asthma, as part of a daily treatment regimen. Cromolyn sodium (Intal) is administered either through an inhaler or a nebulizer and is most effective during periods of stability for an asthmatic child who is known to have frequent exacerbations. It is believed that cromolyn sodium is best at reducing late-stage inflammation. To increase cromolyn sodium's effectiveness, I may prescribe it in conjunction with albuterol (a beta-agonist that opens up the airways).

I believe cromolyn sodium is one of the most useful medications for the treatment of asthma in young children. It's one of my personal favorites because it has so few side effects. My basic regimen is Intal with albuterol if necessary, and the vast majority of my patients get healthier with this prescription.

How Cromolyn Sodium Works

Cromolyn sodium is an anti-inflammatory drug that stabilizes mast cells, which are responsible for starting the inflammatory cascade. Mast cells contain histamine granules, which, when released, cause allergic reactions such as rash, nasal congestion, wheezing, and shortness of breath. In addition, studies have shown that cromolyn sodium significantly inhibits several other inflammatory compounds in the bloodstream, including cytokines. Whether in powder or nebulized form, cromolyn sodium can cause an irritating cough when taken during an acute attack, and for this reason it should not be used in emergencies.

The Most Common Side Effects of Cromolyn Sodium

Cromolyn sodium has few of the side effects of steroids and has been around long enough that most doctors consider it relatively safe. Infrequently, nausea, coughing, drowsiness, and hoarseness can occur.

LEUKOTRIENE INHIBITORS

When Your Doctor May Prescribe Leukotriene Inhibitors

Most doctors prescribe this for patients with mild to moderate asthma when symptoms are present. It is also prescribed for patients with mild intermittent asthma, such as exercise-induced asthma. Leukotriene inhibitors such as Singulair *(montelukast)* or Accolate *(zafirlukast)* seem to prevent attacks in these patients and may prevent the need for steroids. Patients who have not responded to other medications often have success with leukotriene inhibitors. Many doctors consider leukotriene inhibitors a possible first step before considering steroids; other doctors will use them as a second line of treatment after inhaled steroids have proved ineffective.

How Leukotriene Inhibitors Work

A recent breakthrough in asthma research led to the discovery of *leukotrienes,* important chemical messengers that promote inflammation. These inflammatory compounds, which have come into focus as a major contributor to asthma, can lead to airway constriction and mucus production. Leukotrienes have histamine-like qualities and may cause bronchospasms. They also appear to be more potent bronchoconstrictors than histamine. When researchers realized that steroids are ineffective at blocking leukotrienes, the search was on for a drug that could. They eventually developed montelukast (Singulair) and zafirlukast (Accolate), which prevent the body from releasing leukotrienes. These new drugs have been available since 1998 for treating asthma.

Studies have found that there was a significant improvement in peak-flow meter readings and a decreased need for beta-agonists in patients who were on leukotriene inhibitors. Leukotriene inhibitors may also prove useful in combination with other medications, perhaps by reducing the need for them. Current studies are under way to determine the benefit of using leukotriene inhibitors with steroids. A study in the *Archives of Internal Medicine* found that combining Singulair with an antihistamine called *loratadine* over a ten-week period significantly improved asthma control.

The Most Common Side Effects of Leukotriene Inhibitors

So far the drugs appear to be generally well tolerated. There were some initial reports that they elevated liver enzymes, possibly predisposing a patient to liver damage. It is for this reason that some doctors recommend regular blood tests for their patients who are on leukotriene inhibitors. Other side effects include stomachaches, headaches, cold and flu symptoms, itching, and ear and extremity pain.

My biggest concern with these drugs is that they are so new that we really don't know if they have any long-term complications. Some children take asthma drugs for five to ten years, and we just don't have that kind of data on leukotriene inhibitors. A recent article in *Canadian Family Physician* questioned the use of these drugs, saying that they are expensive and not particularly well studied. Indeed, there has been only one study supporting their benefits that lasted longer than one year.

These drugs appear to be effective and may end up being one of the best treatments we have for asthma. Time will tell, just as it has for many asthma medications, what the appropriate role for leukotriene inhibitors will be. Until that point, I believe these drugs should be used cautiously.

BETA-AGONIST SPRAYS (BRONCHODILATORS)

When Your Doctor May Prescribe Beta-Agonist Sprays

These are usually prescribed to be used on an as-needed basis when an attack seems to be coming on, and as a preventive measure before sports for those with exercise-induced asthma. In comparison with other drugs, these are easy to use and immediately effective.

How Beta-Agonist Sprays Work

Beta-agonist sprays open up the airways by attaching to *receptors* on cells in the lung passageway. These beta-2 receptors, once activated, relax constricted lung tissues. All you need is a quick puff and the drug can work for anywhere from one to twelve hours, depending on the brand. For this reason, they are extremely popular, and few asthmatics will leave the house without their reliable spray.

Generally, there are two categories of beta-agonists: *long-acting* and *short-acting*. Both are effective at reducing or preventing symptoms but will not reduce underlying inflammation. Long-acting beta-agonists take more time to kick in than short-acting.

Salmeterol (Serevent), one of the newer long-acting sprays, appears to be useful for children with well-controlled asthma. It has a couple of advantages over its competitors: It appears to be safe when taken with steroids, and it may allow patients to lower their doses of steroids. Salmeterol remains effective for up to twelve hours and is especially useful for children who have trouble getting through the night without wheezing. It takes half an hour to become effective, however, and should not be used in an acute attack.

Short-acting beta-agonist sprays, the most common of which is albuterol (Proventil, Ventolin), are used when symptoms are acute and immediate relief is needed. Some other short-acting beta-agonists that you might have heard of include isoproterenol (Isuprel, Norisodrine, Medihaler-Iso), metaproterenol (Alupent, Metaprel), pirbuterol (Maxair), terbutaline (Brethine, Brethaire, Bricanyl), and bitolterol (Tornalate). Isoetharine (Bronkosol), often prescribed for children in the hospital, lasts only about an hour but is immediately effective and can be used repeatedly throughout the day.

The Most Common Side Effects of Beta-Agonist Sprays

Even though these drugs are designed to target the lungs, there are some beta receptors in the heart as well, and the sprays can lead to an increased heart rate and a drop in blood pressure. Earlier beta-agonist sprays like Alupent were less selective and therefore had more side effects. Other side effects include nervousness, irritability, stomach distress, migraines, and tremors.

Albuterol, the most common short-acting spray, is recommended for children as young as two years old and tends to cause less shakiness than its counterparts. There was a 1995 study that found that albuterol worsened attention deficit disorder in children, but other studies did not support this finding. A promising new short-acting beta-agonist, levalbuterol (Xopenex), appears to be as effective as albuterol but has fewer side effects.

Another downside to beta-agonists is that they become progressively less effective the more they are used. Worse, there is the fear that they exacerbate asthma by exposing the lungs to additional pollution and irritants that could then lead to free-radical damage and ultimately even more inflammation. A study published in the *American Journal of Respiratory and Critical Care Medicine* found that people who were on terbutaline, a common bronchodilating medication, had *increased* levels of inflammatory compounds in their systems and decreased levels of antioxidants, which are crucial in fighting free-radical damage.

A few experts have even suggested that beta-agonists are one of the factors contributing to the worldwide rise in asthma. In Europe between 1961 and 1966, when beta-agonist sprays first became popular, there was a notable jump in the death rate from asthma. Similar patterns have been recorded in the United States. The theory is that beta-agonists mask underlying inflammation of the lungs and may even promote inflammation, and by the time the patient finds them ineffective, he is in such bad shape that nothing seems to work.

THEOPHYLLINE

When Your Doctor May Prescribe Theophylline

When other medications are ineffective. Common brands include Theo-24, Slo-Bid, and Theo-Dur.

How Theophylline Works

While the exact mechanism is unknown, it is believed to work as a bronchodilator. Other research suggests that it works by relaxing the muscles surrounding the bronchial passages.

The Most Common Side Effects of Theophylline

The major problem in the use of theophylline is the need to monitor blood levels for toxicity. Theophylline has a narrow therapeutic range: If it is too low it is ineffective; if it is too high it is toxic. Unfortunately, this means regular blood tests. For this reason, theophylline has fallen out of favor with many physicians and is not used as a first line of treatment.

Side effects include hyperactivity, mood changes, and difficulty concentrating. Some children can't tolerate it at all, though there are many different forms of the drug, and children can switch to another brand if the first is intolerable. I generally do not recommend this drug for children under the age of twelve.

ANTIHISTAMINES

When Your Doctor May Prescribe Antihistamines

Antihistamines are for allergic children during allergy season, in combination with other medications. Antihistamines seem to enhance the effectiveness of leukotriene inhibitors. Many asthmatics are warned not to take antihistamines because of their sedating effects; however, in certain cases antihistamines may prevent an allergic reaction. Antihistamines such as Allegra, Claritin, and Zyrtec are reasonable options for children who have seasonal allergies to pollen and whose symptoms are out of control. I would avoid over-the-counter sedating antihistamines for general allergic symptoms, but there are times when Benadryl or Atarax may be necessary to deal with a severe allergic reaction.

How Antihistamines Work

They block histamine receptors, making the effects of histamine less pronounced.

The Disadvantages of Antihistamines

There is some concern about the rebound effect—that as soon as you stop the antihistamine, the allergic reaction could get worse. Antihistamines can also mask serious underlying problems. If your child is experiencing itchy eyes and a runny nose every morning or evening, every effort should be made to determine the reason why. In short, there is a place for limited use of antihistamines where there is an acute allergic reaction that needs to be stopped.

ADRENALINE

When Your Doctor May Prescribe Adrenaline

This drug is used only in emergency situations. Adrenaline is administered via injection, most often in the form of EpiPen. This small, syringe-like device, when pressed against the skin, automatically injects a predosed amount of medication into a patient. EpiPen is especially important for individuals who have sudden acute asthmatic symptoms and a crisis develops in a matter of minutes. Often these attacks happen as a result of a food allergy. Many parents keep one EpiPen in the car, one in school, and one at home just to make sure there is always one nearby in an emergency.

Generally, one or two well-spaced doses may be necessary. It's best for parents to obtain an EpiPen that is predosed for children. Your doctor may wish to individually dose your child's EpiPen, based on her weight.

In an emergency, adrenaline can save your child's life and can buy time before you get to the emergency room. After administering adrenaline to your child, you should always contact your physician and head to the emergency room. As with all medications, be sure to check expiration dates regularly.

How Adrenaline Works

It opens up the airways immediately and blocks many of the biological processes that occur during anaphylactic shock, such as hypotension, loss of consciousness, edema, bronchoconstriction, and laryngal swelling.

The Most Common Side Effects of Adrenaline

Restlessness, rapid heartbeat, irritability, and nausea.

❧ The Best Sprays for Children ❧

Asthma medications are generally prescribed in one of two ways—with either a *nebulizer* or a *Metered-Dose Inhaler* (MDI). Nebulizers are machines that turn liquid medications into a fine mist, sometimes using ultrasound that is then inhaled. Most nebulizers are relatively inexpensive and come in a variety of sizes, including portable ones. Ultrasonic nebulizers are generally more costly. They are available by prescription.

MDIs are the traditional puffers that most of us are familiar with. You have to be able to press down on the inhaler at the same moment that you take a deep breath. Some children (and adults) have difficulty breathing in and pressing down at the same time. They just can't get the timing right. *Spacers,* tubes that attach to the MDI, are helpful for these people because the mist goes into a chamber, where it remains until the child inhales. No timing is involved, and no coordination is necessary.

Older MDIs use *chlorofluorocarbons* (CFCs) to propel the drug into the lungs. As you no doubt know, CFCs are generally banned throughout the world because they deplete the ozone layer. Inhaler manufacturers were given a special dispensation that allowed them to continue to use CFCs, simply because there wasn't a viable alternative. Now manufacturers have come up with some CFC-free inhalers, including Dry Powder Inhalers (DPIs), with brand names like Diskinhaler and Turbohaler. With a DPI, a small capsule of the drug is emptied into an inhaler device that has a little fan to propel the powder. The advantage to a DPI, especially from a child's point of view, is that it automatically disperses the drug when you inhale. No coordination is necessary. But some of my patients have complained about DPIs and feel they're not as effective as MDIs. Combination medications such as Advair (*fluticasone* and *salmeterol*) also provide a convenient method for treatment.

Always remember to rinse your child's mouth out after using an inhaler device. This will prevent medication from being swallowed into the body and minimize the risk of thrush or other side effects.

How to Get Your Child Off Steroids

First, never suddenly stop taking oral steroids. Sudden cessation can cause significant organ damage and may also lead to a life-threatening condition called *adrenal failure*. This happens when the adrenal gland, which sits above the kidney and is crucial for producing the body's natural steroids, actually shuts down, leaving the body vulnerable to a variety of illnesses.

Before weaning your child off steroids, always discuss a dosage regimen with your physician and make sure she monitors your child's progress. The following are general guidelines that I use in my practice, but every doctor may have slight variations. Depending on the age of the child, I may start with a dose as high as 30 milligrams a day. I then reduce this dose by 5–10 milligrams per day or every other day, depending on the severity of the child's problem. For inhaled steroids, I advise that patients decrease the number of puffs from four to three to two to one to zero, either every day or every other day. I may also extend these reduction programs into a week to two weeks of therapy, depending on whether symptoms have abated. Translation: If your child is still wheezing and her peak-flow numbers are still low, this is not the appropriate time to reduce drugs or switch off the steroids. Depending on the patient, the severity of symptoms, and the amount of time the patient has been on steroids, a steroid-reduction program is done over a period of days or weeks and occasionally months.

Most doctors find that reducing steroids is easier than going off them entirely. Certainly, getting off steroids when a child has been on them for a long time is a difficult process. Again, your doctor can help.

WHAT ARE RECOMMENDED DOSES FOR CHILDREN?

Below are some broad dosage guidelines for asthma drugs and children. Of course, the intent of the Breath of Life program is to provide parents with an overview of natural treatments for asthma. But everyone should have a general sense of what to expect when the doctor prescribes drugs for his child. Every child is different, and any dosages should be discussed and monitored by your child's doctor.

- **Steroids:** In the 1960s, when steroids were first put on the market, these drugs were routinely prescribed in doses of 100 to 200 milligrams per day. Now the generally recommended starting dose of Prednisone (an oral steroid) for children is usually between 5 and 30 milligrams per day, usually to be tapered off during the following one to two weeks after an attack.

There are dozens of options for inhaled steroids. Hence, it's impossible to give general guidelines. Just as an example, a doctor might recommend two puffs a day of Flovent 44-microgram spray for a month to six weeks after an acute attack. Or he or she may recommend that your child stay on this dose for many months or even years. Many steroids are not recommended for very young children; budesonide, for instance, is not recommended for children under age six. Your doctor will know the age limit for any drug that she recommends. Generally, weaning off of medications takes time and should be done cautiously.

· **Beta-Agonist (Bronchodilator) Sprays:** Again, these sprays come in many brands and in many different strengths. I find that two to four puffs a day of Proventil (albuterol), or once or twice a day by nebulizer, or one to two puffs twice a day of Serevent (a newer, long-acting bronchodilator) is effective. Proventil is not recommended for children under two; Serevent is not recommended for children under six. These medicines are available for a nebulizer as well.

· **Cromolyn Sodium:** Between two to eight inhalations per day from an inhaler, or one to two nebulizer treatments per day.

· **Leukotriene-Receptor Inhibitors:** Five to 10 mg at bedtime. Singulair is not recommended for children under age two. Accolate is not for children under six.

· **Antihistamines:** Allegra and Claritin are not recommended for children under six, but Zyrtec and Benadryl can be taken by children as young as two. In certain situations, a physician may recommend Benadryl.

• **Adrenaline:** Via EpiPen or by a formula of 0.01 milliliters of adrenaline multiplied by the child's weight in kilograms.

How to Use a Peak-Flow Meter

The best way for parents to track their child's asthma is to use a peak-flow meter, a simple tube-shaped device. Peak-flow meters are one of the most important tools we have for monitoring an asthmatic's condition at home and for checking the effectiveness of his medication. A peak-flow meter is one of the most reliable at-home tools to monitor your child's daily progress. It can be used both before and after your child takes his or her medication, or every day. Peak-flow meters are available through prescription.

To use a peak-flow meter, your child takes a deep breath, creates a seal with his lips over the opening of the tube, and blows as forcefully as he can. The device then measures the amount of air exhaled in the first second. For asthmatics, this is the period when problems are most detectable. The results of the first reading are noted, either by a marker on the peak-flow meter or on a piece of paper. The process is repeated again and recorded. The average or the higher of the two results is noted on their daily record.

Some children—especially those younger than five—have a hard time handling these devices. Even some adults have problems. It's not a matter of coordination or intelligence; for some people, it's just not comfortable. Once your child gets the hang of it, though, you will have a helpful tool in monitoring her ongoing status. Record your child's peak-flow reading every morning and evening, and monitor the numbers in the booklet that usually comes with the peak-flow meter. If your child is old enough, give her a clipboard and some graph paper to chart her own progress. Soon both of you will begin to recognize a pattern.

Let's say, for instance, that the consistent reading on the peak-flow meter is 200 cubic meters per second. While meter scales may vary, a drop of 10 percent is significant; a 30 to 50 percent drop is usually considered critical. Bear in mind, though, that different people have different thresholds. Some patients drop 10 percent and have serious symptoms; others drop 30 percent and feel only minimal tightness. There's no exact ratio. This is why you need regular peak-flow meter readings to identify the danger zone for your child. Doctors have more sophisticated ways to measure the progress of your child's recovery, including a pulmonary function test, which evaluates several aspects of a patient's total lung capacity, including both the large and small airways. It's helpful to present your peak-flow meter results to your physician so he can compare it to his results. This will give you and your doctor the most accurate picture of your child's health.

chapter six

Nutritional Healing

We all know how fickle kids are at the dinner table. As hard as you try to get your children to eat right, it's difficult to make sure they get the nutrients they need through diet alone. I've worked with enough asthmatic kids to know that adding nutritional supplements can go a long way toward getting them healthy.

There are plenty of skeptics who don't believe supplements can help people with asthma. And I agree that more research is vital to increase our understanding of the power and risks of the many substances found in nutritional supplements. But supplements aren't just a fad. Consider folic acid. If a pregnant woman consumes enough folic acid (a common B vitamin), according to a 1995 study in the *Lancet,* the risk of her baby developing *spina bifida* is reduced to almost zero. The role of B vitamins in preventing cardiovascular disease is now recognized. Calcium can prevent osteoporosis.

As you will read below, I also believe that enough data have come in to support the use of nutritional supplements in the treatment of asthma.

In my experience, I have found that children are very responsive to supplements and that their lungs are so receptive that adding nutrients to their diet or improving their diets makes a huge difference. I have watched patients take supplements and regain their health. If my experience is any guide, we are going to find that certain supplements are very powerful treatments for many people. Bear in mind, however, that too many supplements can be harmful and there is no excuse for overdosing.

Kelly was a twelve-year-old girl who loved soccer. When I first saw her in my office, she told me that she would find herself short of breath on and off the field. She didn't always have the stamina for an entire game and often relied on her inhalers. Kelly frequently got colds and had already had to miss several games of the season when she came to me. I started her on vitamin C and magnesium. At the first sign of a cold, I instructed her to use echinacea, an herbal remedy often prescribed in Europe that's thought to stimulate the immune system. I also helped her to begin working on all aspects of the Breath of Life program. By the end of the season, Kelly was able to play through the games, had reduced her asthma medications by half, and had stopped getting sick. She did so well that the following year she was elected captain of the team.

Many people use the words *vitamin* and *supplement* interchangeably. Technically, this is inaccurate. Supplements can be broken down into vitamins, minerals, amino acids, fatty acids, and a host of other compounds, including bioflavonoids and isoflavones. I describe these in detail in my book *The Nutraceutical Revolution* (Riverhead Books, 1999).

Below I will focus on the relatively small army of researched nutrients that can help to heal asthma. When I believe supplements are appropriate, I often start with an antioxidant such as vitamin C and the mineral magnesium. Other nutrients that I may prescribe for children include a general multivitamin or antioxidant formula, N-acetyl-L-cysteine (NAC), selenium, zinc, and omega-3 fatty acids or fish oils. As you will see below, there is an accumulating body of research indicating that people with the highest intake of these anti-asthma nutrients have the lowest rates of asthma.

Do not make the mistake of thinking that more is better. I see many people who take high doses of supplements randomly and think this will be the route to good health. But some supplements in high doses can have adverse effects, including gastric irritation or reflux. Excess vitamin C has been linked to kidney stones, and overdoses of magnesium can cause diarrhea. **A well-balanced group of supplements should be taken under the guidance of a physician, and your doctor must be aware of any supplements that your child is taking.** Then you can be alerted to any potential interactions with other supplements or medications. The doses I suggest below are a general guideline and should be discussed with your doctor. They may be higher or lower depending on a child's specific needs. Supplements should be consumed in an age-appropriate form. Therefore powders, tinctures, and chewable tablets may be more suitable for very young children, and capsules, tablets, and gels may be better for children over the age of ten.

It's also important to remember that supplements do not replace drugs. Without exception, supplements should not be used in place of medication during an acute attack. In general, acute or life-threatening symptoms of asthma should be treated with medications. Supplements should be taken to prevent acute attacks from happening in the first place, to complement medical therapy, and to promote healing. (For specific information on supplements or other issues, visit Ask the Doctor at www.drcity.com.)

MAGNESIUM

One of the most popular supplements for asthmatics is the mineral magnesium. There is tantalizing research showing that magnesium—when added to nebulized albuterol—leads to improved pulmonary function. Many researchers are investigating its use with a variety of different approaches. In addition to oral magnesium, many hospitals supplement asthma medications with intravenous magnesium for an acute attack in teenagers and adults. One theory as to why magnesium works is that it relaxes the muscles surrounding the bronchial tubes.

A number of recent studies have revealed magnesium's effectiveness. A study in *The European Respiratory Journal* found that nebulized magnesium, when used to treat acute asthma, had a bronchodilatory effect similar to that of nebulized salbutamol, a bronchodilator. Other studies have concluded that there seemed to be a correlation between low levels of magnesium and airway hyper-responsiveness in asthmatic patients. *The Journal of Family Practice* reported that the higher rates of illness in African-Americans in urban areas may be due to a lack of magnesium. A recent study supported the practice of adding magnesium to other medications for asthma patients with acute symptoms or who end up in the emergency room. *Thorax* recently reported that deficiencies in vitamins A, C, E, and magnesium were associated with more severe symptoms in patients with *brittle asthma* (a rare form of asthma). In short, there is a significant body of evidence that magnesium plays an important role in asthma.

Jack, a seven-year-old patient of mine, was having constant flare-ups of his asthma. His parents made significant progress by incorporating the Breath of Life program in his life—monitoring the foods he was eating, making sure his bedroom was free of dust mites, and so forth. Still, his asthma continued to flare up from time to time. I started him on a regimen of 200 milligrams of magnesium a day, and his mother was amazed to see that he started to feel better. The magnesium had a noticeable impact on his health and put him a step closer to recovery. He had a reduced need for his albuterol inhaler, and he responded better to it when he did need it. Here's an example of a child who had a significant and almost immediate response after being put on very simple sup-plementation. His condition continued to improve as he stuck to the principles of the Breath of Life program.

Magnesium can sometimes cause diarrhea, cramps, or other abdominal complaints. If your child experiences this, discontinue the supplement immediately. In certain situations, your doctor may recommend a red blood cell magnesium test to determine if a magnesium deficiency exists. My suggested daily dose of magnesium for asthmatic children is as follows:

- Kids from two to four years old—up to 100 milligrams
- Kids from five to ten—up to 200 milligrams
- Kids from ten to fifteen—200–500 milligrams

VITAMIN C

Vitamin C is a powerful antioxidant that can disarm free radicals (for more on antioxidants, see "What Are Free Radicals?" on page 88). A recent report suggests that pulmonary tissue can be damaged in many ways by chemicals and pesticides and that antioxidants can help prevent and repair this damage. Vitamin C may have other positive properties as well. Research suggests that it is anti-inflammatory, decreases the risk of respiratory infection, and has some natural antihistamine effects. As early as 1994, the *Annals of Allergy* reported that vitamin C was beneficial in treating asthma and allergies. Since then, studies have rolled in endorsing this conclusion: British researchers found that the reduced intake of antioxidants, including vitamin C, in the British diet of the past twenty-five years has probably contributed to the increase in the prevalence of asthma. Last year, *The Journal of Asthma* reported that "decreased antioxidant protection may contribute to the pathogenesis of mild asthma."

An interesting recent study from the *Lancet* indicates that in order to gain the maximum benefits of vitamin C, it is necessary to saturate the lungs with vitamins and that simple blood tests may not give us the true picture. The body will try to maintain normal levels of vitamin C in the blood, while the lung lining itself is starved for the nutrient. Therefore, an asthmatic child may need higher levels than others.

I generally recommend that asthmatic children who are experiencing chronic symptoms start on the doses mentioned below, then reduce them by as much as half once they are stronger and healthier. Vitamin C is part of an overall program, and often adequate amounts can be ingested through the diet. Again, a doctor should monitor these doses.

My suggested daily dose for asthmatic children with moderate to severe asthma:

- Kids from two to four years old—50 to 100 milligrams
- Kids from five to ten—up to 250 milligrams
- Kids from ten to fifteen—up to 500 milligrams

SELENIUM AND NAC

These nutrients help the body produce *glutathione,* one of the most powerful free-radical fighters produced by the body. Glutathione is crucial in protecting the body from destructive by-products of many chronic illnesses, including asthma. It is found throughout the body but in higher levels in the lungs and the liver. Studies have confirmed that individuals with chronic medical conditions such as asthma have lower levels of glutathione. *Food and Chemical Toxicology* reported in 1999 that glutathione may act as an antioxidant for the lungs.

Glutathione is a wonderful compound, but glutathione supplements rapidly disintegrate once they are absorbed into the body. Supplements that can increase the body's natural production of glutathione are essential. One of these is N-Acetyl-1 Cysteine (NAC), which may help stimulate the body's natural production of glutathione. NAC has also been shown to thin and reduce mucus.

Another nutrient that helps to stimulate glutathione production is *selenium,* one of the ten essential trace minerals. Selenium also helps vitamin E quench free radicals. Asthmatics tend to have low levels of selenium. In 1990, *Thorax* published a study that found a nearly sixfold increase in the risk of asthma in New Zealand patients with low levels of selenium. Another study in 1993 showed that patients with more selenium in their bloodstream had less pulmonary inflammation. Low levels of selenium have also been linked to a higher risk for cancer.

My suggested daily dose of NAC for asthmatic children:

- Kids from two to four years old—100 milligrams
- Kids from five to ten—up to 250 milligrams
- Kids from ten to fifteen—up to 500 milligrams

My suggested daily dose of selenium for asthmatic children:

- Kids from two to four years old—up to 50 micrograms
- Kids from five to ten—50 to 100 micrograms
- Kids from ten to fifteen—100 to 200 micrograms

ZINC

According to a study done in 1996, patients with asthma have less zinc in their blood than do healthy people. Zinc has been a popular supplement ever since a study at the Cleveland Clinic indicated that it prevented the common cold. Further studies have failed to replicate this finding, but many of my patients report that taking zinc when they feel a cold coming on is helpful. Cold viruses can stimulate a number of responses, including constriction of airways and increased mucus production, and can ultimately provoke an asthma attack. If zinc prevents colds or increases resistance, then this can be a great benefit for an asthmatic.

One patient comes to mind that had great success with zinc. Four-year-old Caitlin regularly caught colds from her preschool *germ exchange,* which would then lead to constant flare-ups of her asthma. The next school season, when Caitlin was five, I put her on a low dose of zinc, as well as echinacea and goldenseal, two popular herbal cold remedies. The occurrence of colds and respiratory problems was significantly reduced, which calmed down Caitlin's asthma. One note for parents is that herbal products should not be taken for longer than six weeks unless recommended by your physician.

I recommend that asthmatic children take zinc only during cold and flu season, or when you detect a cold coming on. My suggested daily dose during these times is:

- Kids from two to four years old—5 milligrams
- Kids from five to ten—up to 10 milligrams
- Kids from ten to 15—up to 20 milligrams

Omega-3 Fatty Acids

Another star in the nutritional arsenal, omega-3 fatty acids are essential anti-inflammatory compounds that may help prevent asthma. Fish oils contain two essential fatty acids, *docosahexanoic acid* (DHA) and *eicosapentenoic acid* (EPA). Similar to leukotriene-inhibiting medications, fish oils slow down inflammation and promote the production of helpful prostaglandins that regulate the body's inflammatory processes. The current uncertainty about fish oil is whether it's useful when taken for only a short period of time.

Omega-3s are considered essential fatty acids because the body cannot manufacture these acids itself. Yet there are limited numbers of foods that provide these acids; these include fish or flaxseed oil. The essential fatty acids found in fish oil are in a more usable form than those in flaxseed oil, which need several enzymes in the body to make them effective. Ideally you'll serve your kids more fish, and you can even combine flaxseed oil with other healthy oils, such as olive oil in your salad dressing. But it may be necessary to add fish oil capsules to your kids' diet. These oils offer a gentle treatment that slowly, over time, may help the body repair tissue damage.

In the event that it is necessary to add more fish oil to your child's diet, supplements are available, though be forewarned that fish oil supplements do have a fishy taste. Check the date on the bottle to ensure that the supplements are as fresh as possible, since oils can become rancid over time, reducing their effectiveness.

My suggested daily dose of fish oil or flaxseed oil capsules for asthmatic children:

- Kids from two to four years old—up to 100 milligrams
- Kids from five to ten—250 to 500 milligrams
- Kids from ten to fifteen—500 to 1,000 milligrams

QUERCETIN AND STINGING NETTLE

With so many asthmatic children suffering from allergies, I regularly turn to two allergy-fighting nutrients: *quercetin* and *stinging nettle*. Quercetin is a bioflavonoid that is primarily known for the blue and red color it gives to plants. It appears to be an anti-inflammatory as well as an antihistamine. It stops allergic reactions by preventing mast cell degranulation, which prevents histamines and a host of other inflammatory compounds from being released into the bloodstream.

Stinging nettle, a common annoyance in nearly every garden, can also help to dampen allergies. Despite the fact that they burn your skin when you brush up against them in your yard, nettle leaves have been shown to possess anti-inflammatory properties. They prevent the body from making inflammatory prostaglandins and work like a natural antihistamine. Nettles contain more than twenty-four different chemical components, from vitamins to proteins to flavonoids. One study found that of sixty-nine people with hay fever, 57 percent had a major improvement in their symptoms after taking nettles.

I usually recommend that children take these supplements only when they are at risk for allergies, such as during pollen season. Generally, patients take them for only a few weeks at a time.

My suggested daily dose of quercetin for asthmatic children:

- Kids from two to four years old—200 milligrams
- Kids from five to ten—400 milligrams
- Kids from ten to fifteen—600 milligrams

My suggested daily dose of stinging nettles for asthmatic children:

- Kids from two to four years old—200 milligrams
- Kids from five to ten—400 milligrams
- Kids from ten to fifteen—800 milligrams

~ What Are Free Radicals? ~

Name a major disease, and it's a pretty good bet that free radicals are involved. Cancer, cardiovascular disease, diabetes, and yes, asthma, can point a finger of blame at these highly volatile molecules.

Free radicals are basically molecules missing a part. Normally every atom has paired electrons. When an atom contains an extra electron or is deficient in an electron, it has unpaired electrons and can then be considered a free radical. These unpaired electrons, in a crazy desire to find a match, bounce around to neighboring molecules until they can steal an electron. Free radicals are natural; in fact, they are a crucial part of our own immune defenses. Our bodies use free radicals to kill viruses and bacteria, and they are a normal by-product of our everyday metabolism.

When our bodies have more than they can handle, however, free radicals start to swipe electrons from the cells of our healthy tissues. This is when free-radical damage occurs. Healthy cells that lose an electron can then contain free radicals themselves, and thus begins a chain reaction that can continue indefinitely.

What causes free radicals? We are exposed to molecules—from air pollution, smoking, chemical fumes—that are either free radicals themselves or that create free radicals once they enter our bodies. Ozone contains an unpaired electron, for instance. If you inhale ozone, it can damage healthy cells through its attempt to find a match. Junk food, with its high quantities of hydrogenated fats and sugar, tends to promote free-radical damage.

Our bodies have some natural defenses against excessive free radicals, specific compounds called *antioxidants,* which serve as electron donors. By donating an electron to the free radical, antioxidants are able to stop the chain reaction in its tracks, rendering the molecules harmless before they cause damage. We end up with a free-radical overload when we exercise, for instance, but our bodies are usually able to cope with this temporary overload on their own. It is when we suffer repeated free-radical invasions—from air pollution, a high-fat diet, exposure to toxins like asbestos—that we get into trouble.

That's why we need to have a diet high in antioxidants, which can help to mop up excess free radicals. The best antioxidants include vitamins A, C, and E, selenium, and zinc. Vitamin A belongs to a family of compounds called *carotenoids*. Remember that popping vitamin C pills with every meal won't necessarily do the trick. Some vitamins, when taken in excessive doses, can be dangerous.

It's important to take a full regimen of antioxidants. A doctor or nutritionist can help you make sure you take in the right combination of antioxidants. These compounds work together, and each has a specific function. When vitamin E has mopped up as many free radicals as it can hold, for instance, vitamin C carts them away, freeing vitamin E up to continue its work. In addition, different antioxidants help support different areas of the body. Vitamin E works in the fatty part of cells, while vitamin C is water-soluble, so it works best in the liquid portion of cells, including the fluid lining in the lungs. For this reason, vitamin C appears to have a crucial role for asthmatics.

What are the best food sources for antioxidants? Fruits, vegetables, nuts, seeds, and whole grains. Vitamin C is found in fruits and vegetables, vitamin E is found in grains, and carotenoids are found in yellow vegetables like squash and carrots. Many nuts and seeds contain selenium and zinc. Supplements are another good source of antioxidants but should be considered as exactly what their name implies: an additive to a healthy diet.

CALCIUM

Asthmatics have a higher risk of osteoporosis, for several reasons. They tend to exercise less than they should, and they take steroids, which can contribute to bone loss. Even inhaled steroids may increase the risk for osteoporosis. Further, children who are lactose-intolerant or allergic to milk are at an even bigger disadvantage because they don't consume enough bone-building calcium. For these reasons, I generally recommend that asthmatic children take calcium supplements.

My suggested daily dose of calcium for asthmatic children:

- Kids from two to four years old—100 milligrams
- Kids from five to ten—250 milligrams
- Kids from ten to fifteen—500 milligrams

HERBS AND OTHER MEDICINAL PLANTS

For centuries herbs have been used as medicines. Today, over 75% of the world's population uses herbs as one of their primary treatments. In general, herbs are safer than many medications. That is not to say that pharmaceuticals are dangerous or that, in many cases, they won't provide more prompt relief than alternative measures. However, herbs, just like medicines, have side effects, and should be used with caution, especially in the case of children or pregnant women. In addition, because of possible chemical interactions, herbs should be taken with medication only under the direct supervision of your child's physician. For example, we know that herbs such as St. John's Wort may decrease the effectiveness of certain drugs, and that Ginkgo may increase bleeding time, particularly in individuals taking aspirin or anticoagulants.

Which herbs are the best choice for your child will depend on their age, preference, and the ease with which they can be administered. I do not recommend herbs for every child—each case should be assessed on an individual basis. Just as with medication, herbs should be consumed in moderation—more is definitely not better—and dosages should be adjusted by weight or age. Unlike vitamins, herbs should not be consumed on a daily basis, but rather for a periodic and strictly defined amount of time. Also remember that results will vary depending on the quality of the herbs. When possible, choose organic herb sources. Parents should also look for signs of allergy or toxicity such as diarrhea, vomiting, cramps or irritability if their children are given herbs. **Most importantly, herbal supplements are not recommended for children under the age of ten unless prescribed by your child's physician.**

Herbs come in several forms, the most common being capsules and tincture extracts, which are available alcohol-free. Whenever capsules are used, a standardized form of the herb is recommended; however, in general, I find tinctures most useful for children. Parents can even add a tincture to a child's favorite juice to make it easier to consume.

As with the other nutrients, the herbs that may be used in treating asthma fall into three basic categories: anti-inflammatories, bronchodilators, and antihistamines.

Ginkgo

Ginkgo, one of the most famous Chinese herbs, has long been prescribed for allergies in traditional Chinese medicine. This herb contains flavonglycosides, proanthocyanadins, and terpenes, and has been proven to increase circulation throughout the body and inhibit PAF (platelet-activating-factor) in the blood stream. PAF occurs when there is inflammation in the body, and can be a potent trigger of allergies. The use of ginkgo, along with fish oils, mentioned earlier, can help to ease allergies and asthma. Ginkgo should be taken as a standardized extract of 24 percent.

Feverfew

Feverfew, officially known as *Tanacetum parthenium,* contains two powerful plant chemicals known as parthenolide and sesquiterpenes, and first became famous for its ability to ease migraines. Like the chemicals in ginkgo, the parthenolide in feverfew has been shown to inhibit PAF, prostaglandins, and histamine—all of which are associated with inflammation.

Coleus Forskohlii

This herb is well known in Indian Ayurvedic medicine. The active ingredient, forskolin, helps increase compounds in the body that relax bronchial muscles. Double-blind studies have shown that the herb is as effective as the drug fenoterol, a bronchodilator, without the side effects of shakiness and tremors. Standardized extracts of the herb are most effective if they contain 18 percent forskolin.

Ginger

Ginger is known to have potent anti-inflammatory properties, as well as providing a soothing effect on sore throats and settling upset tummies. As with most herbal remedies, I prefer ginger in herbal tincture form or teas. Fresh ginger can be sliced, simmered for about twenty minutes in water, and sweetened with honey.

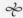

Licorice

This is an extensively studied herb whose formal name is *Glycyrrhiza glabra*. It contains antiallergic, antibacterial, and anti-inflammatory compounds. Two of its components have cortisol-like effects in the body. There is one ingredient in licorice that can raise blood pressure, but deglycyrrhizinated commercial products eliminate this problem. DGL (deglycyrrhizinated licorice) is available as a powder, chewable tablet, or tincture. For children I recommend licorice in tea form.

Echinacea

One of the most studied herbs in the world, Echinacea (purple coneflower) is anti-infective, antibacterial, and antiviral. The herb stimulates our immune system's B-cells and T-cells and aids in tissue regeneration. It is generally not recommended before the age of two.

Above is a brief overview of the most common herbs and medicinal plants that I often use to supplement a child's asthma nutrient program. In my practice, I specify the dosage and how long each child should take a particular herb. Review this information with your doctor if you want to start your child on any of the above recommended herbal treatments for asthma. Remember that herbs should only be used to treat children under the direct supervision of their physician.

chapter seven

Catching Your Breath

The breathing exercises discussed below can help your child strengthen his lung muscles, learn how to breathe deeply, and reduce anxiety. Breathing deeply has other benefits: It increases concentration, creativity, and learning ability, as well as energy and alertness. The word *inspiration,* in fact, is derived from the Latin word *inspirare,* which means to breathe in or infuse.

After you and your child become adept at the breathing lessons, you can rely on them to halt the panic that often accompanies an asthma attack. One of the most troubling aspects of asthma is fear: The child who is terrified that she can't breathe and the parent who fears that his child won't make it. Breathing is one of the few body responses that we have some control over. Most of our body systems are on automatic pilot; we have no direct control over our digestion, blood flow, or chemical reactions. This automatic pilot is called the *autonomic nervous system.* While we certainly can't stop ourselves from breathing, we can slow our breathing down and speed it up. Just as Lamaze exercises help parents through childbirth, the Breath of Life breathing routine helps both the asthma sufferer and the parents to relax and calm down during an episode.

The Breath of Life breathing skills also encourage your child to think about the positive power of air and the beauty it can provide. Your asthmatic child is at a difficult crossroads in life. At a time when his relationship with the external environment is being formed, he is learning—as early as preschool—that the polluted air he breathes could be the very reason he has asthma. If you begin now, you can decrease distrust and fearfulness and reframe his attitude toward breathing, relaxation, and enjoyment of air.

With the younger kids in my practice, for example, I talk about the tides and waves, windmills powering electricity, panthers running, tigers jumping, and butterflies fluttering. All because of air. I ask the children to draw a picture of what air can do, and they hand me pictures of airplanes, balloons, birds, and clouds moving across the sky. Instead of feeling threatened, these children learn how important air is to them and the world around them.

To start, you'll want to explain to your child the importance of alignment. Have him lie down on a blanket or soft mat on the floor. Then help him become aware of what it feels like when his spine is relaxed and flat on the floor. One way to do this is to see if you can gently slip your hand between his back and the floor. Initially there may be an upward curve in the lower part of his spine and his shoulders may be slightly raised, but as he becomes aware of this he can gently relax them against the floor. Ask him to notice how his rib cage is positioned when his spine is straight.

It is very important for your child to experience the sensation of feeling totally relaxed while breathing. This is like setting a solid foundation for anything the child needs to do. Our bodies, minds, and emotions function at their freest and best when we are fundamentally relaxed. Encourage this relaxation by doing a body check: Ask if her face is relaxed, then her shoulders, arms, fingers, chest, stomach, legs, feet, and toes. Help her to get a sense of how relaxing it is to let the floor support her— she doesn't have to do anything except relax and rest there. Tell her to imagine she is lying on a magic carpet and the carpet can take her wherever she would like to go. Or tell her to imagine that she is resting on a soft, billowy cloud.

During the first few sessions, you might want to reverse roles with your child, with you lying down and your child checking to see if your spine and shoulders are relaxed. Make a game of it by slightly raising one shoulder to see if he catches you and truly understands how he should lie on the floor when it's his turn. Children learn very quickly, so each time they lie down, you will find that they can relax more quickly and more spontaneously than before. Relaxation will become a remembered experience, and your child will become more and more adept at re-creating that sense of peace and tranquillity, giving him a sense of confidence and control. This is a skill we have when we are born but that we can easily forget as we grow older and engage in life's challenges.

Playing soothing music while you're doing the lessons is helpful for some people and can often make children more willing to do them regularly. With younger children, you may want to invest in a stethoscope to make the exercises more playful. Your child can listen to her heartbeat and lungs while breathing. It's also helpful to know how your child's lungs sound when she's healthy and how they sound when she's wheezing. Your doctor can instruct you on how to use one.

Older children will have no trouble learning the routine, and after the first few sessions will probably want to do it on their own. They will also probably want to skip the last three lessons, as they are designed for younger kids.

Parents will want to do all the following breathing routines with younger children, however. I know how hard it is, during your busy day, to stop and literally catch your breath. But this takes only minutes a day, and it is important for your child to know you are doing this together. Try setting aside the same time each day. After dinner or before bedtime is good; even mornings are okay.

If your child doesn't want to do the breathing on a particular day, don't make a big deal of it. Instead, use the time to talk and connect with your child. A lot of parents tell me that these discussions are wonderfully helpful. With younger children especially, you can talk about how breathing well can help reduce your child's symptoms and allow him to do more of the things he likes to do. You can meditate together or do some visualization, perhaps incorporating a favorite bedtime story or after-school activity (see Chapter 8 for more on visualization techniques). The point is to somehow get across the idea that breathing and relaxing are very important. Eventually, they always get it.

BREATH OF LIFE BREATHING ROUTINE

Belly Breathing

This is the basic exercise that is the foundation for good breathing. Instruct your child to lie on her back, either on a mat or a bed, with her legs bent or straight. Ask her to breathe in through her nose, feeling the breath going into the back of her throat. Or have your child imagine that the air is going in through her belly button and out through her belly button. Make sure the top of her chest is as motionless as possible. Ask her to keep her upper body still and to use her belly muscles to force out the air so that her stomach collapses. When she breathes in, tell her to expand her stomach as far as she can.

Parents can count while the child is breathing: inhale for four counts, exhale for five. Then go up to six counts in for every seven counts out. You'll notice that breathing in takes fewer counts than breathing out, which is normal. A major problem for asthmatics is exhalation, because air gets trapped in the lungs. It's this trapped air that makes breathing in difficult.

Belly-Breathing Variations

Kids might want to belly-breathe with an object on their stomachs. You can use a book, a Game Boy, a stuffed animal, or any treasured object. The idea is to make the toy rise when you breathe in and fall when you breathe out. The object will help accentuate the breathing as well as build up abdominal muscles.

Take the object off and have your child draw his knees to his chest when he exhales, pushing all the air out of his lungs, and bring his legs back to the floor when he inhales, filling his belly with air. Have your kid stand up and swing his arms one way for inhalation, another way for exhalation.

Eventually your child can do belly breathing whenever he has downtime. With his shoulders relaxed and his hands on his stomach, with each fingertip of each hand touching, he can inhale so that his hands separate, then exhale so they come together again.

The Bellows

This will help your child exhale completely to make way for new air. Children need to understand that before you can get clean new air into your lungs, you must get rid of the stale old air. You can illustrate this by showing them a full glass of water and seeing if they can pour any more water in. Only after you pour the old water out is there room for new water.

Have your child sit in a chair and do belly breathing. As he exhales, he can slowly start to lean forward from the waist. Ask him to pull in his stomach as he does so. He can continue to exhale until his head is close to his knees. Now have him purse his lips so that he makes a hissing sound as he pulls in his stomach even tighter and exhales every last drop of air. If your child blows out with pursed lips (as if blowing out a candle), this creates a subtle back pressure that helps to open airways and strengthen the diaphragm. Now have him begin to take a belly breath, inhaling slowly and rising from the waist so that by the time he is sitting up again, his lungs are filled with fresh air.

Have him lean forward again, but this time as quickly as he can, and have him suck in his stomach as if he's just been punched. Ask him to breathe out all the air and then make a hissing sound until his lungs are empty. Then have him relax and sit up slowly, inhaling.

Heart Breathing

This is a good exercise to help your child understand the mind-body connection and to realize that a good attitude and self-confidence can actually help improve asthma. By eliminating panic and remaining in a calm state, many asthma attacks do not become serious. This exercise requires a stethoscope, unless your child is old enough to feel her pulse and count. You may want to spend the first few sessions just having your child listen and count her heartbeats. Then have her belly-breathe and listen to her heart. For every seven beats, breathe in. For every nine beats, breathe out. She'll hear her heart slow down. Now have her breathe shallow and fast, and she'll hear her heart speed up. When she starts to have an asthma attack or gets scared, that's how her heartbeat speeds up. By breathing deeply and relaxing, your child can slow her pulse down and possibly prevent an asthma attack from becoming serious.

Blowing the Sailboat

Ask your child to imagine he is moving a little sailboat along the water on a lovely summer's day. Inhale and exhale, gently blowing the boat's sails. Move the boat from one shore to the other. This is a good one to do with your child before he goes to sleep, and the "shore" can be either side of the bed. Or it can be done with a real sailboat in the bath. The idea here is to have your child blow air out in a steady stream.

Blowing Bubbles

Get a small bottle of bubbles and see who can blow the biggest bubble. Try to keep it in the air as long as possible. Instruct your child to blow the bubble as slowly as possible. See who keeps the bubble up the longest. Then you can blow many bubbles at once and ask your child to make them dance by blowing them up or down. The point of the exercise is to extend his breaths for as long as possible and gain control over his breathing. A variation on this exercise is to use pinwheels on sticks and see who can keep them spinning the longest.

Chest Stretch

This will help open up the entire chest. Ask your child to stand with his feet at shoulders' width, with his shoulders relaxed and his arms dangling by his sides. Tell him to inhale while stretching his head back as far as possible. On exhalation, he lowers his head, leaning forward from the waist, slowly pulling his stomach in until the tips of his fingers touch the floor. Then he can stay there for a moment and gradually return to an upright position

For illustrations of many of the above breathing exercises, visit www. drcity.com/conditions/breathing_corr.shtml.

❧ How to Breathe ❧

Most people breathe shallowly, with their shoulders slumped forward, restricting the expansion of the lungs. When they're asked to take a deep breath, their shoulders go up and their chest goes out, mimicking military posture. This is the worst possible posture for asthmatics.

Instead, you should teach your child *diaphragmatic breathing,* to breathe with his back straight, shoulders relaxed, and abdomen slightly pulled in. Diaphragmatic breathing ultimately increases the amount of oxygen that you take in, slowing down your heart rate and reducing the panic that is often associated with asthma attacks. Knowing how to do these breathing exercises increases the likelihood that panic will be under control.

Ask your child to picture his lungs as two air sacs sitting on top of the diaphragm, the strong horizontal muscle between the lungs and the stomach that is responsible for drawing in every breath of air we take. Without the help of this muscle, we can never truly take a deep breath. The lungs are protected by the rib cage, which is designed to expand freely when air is inhaled and return to resting position on exhalation. The best way to utilize all the available lung space when you inhale is to imagine you are gradually filling up the lower portion of the lungs first, then the middle section, and then the top. While you are doing this, expand your stomach, which will draw the diaphragm muscle down and provide more space for the lungs. To exhale, imagine the above sequence reversed: Draw in the belly to push up the diaphragm muscle, which will cause the lungs to expel the air. By making sure all the air is expelled, you will ensure that the reflex action of inhalation comes naturally.

chapter eight

Mind over Matter

It's no secret that our minds are much more powerful than we recognize. Gurus and spiritual healers know that the mind can have a powerful effect on our health, on how we feel, and on how we act. In Western medicine, doctors have long been aware of this as well. The *placebo effect,* when a person responds to a sugar pill as if it were a medication, is well established. The placebo response can be elicited not just when a patient thinks he is taking a medicine but also when he is treated compassionately. The word *placebo,* in fact, entered our vocabulary as a phrase meaning to please rather than to benefit. While HMOs might not agree, a compassionate physician goes a long way toward healing a patient.

The idea that we can heal our bodies through our minds is even explored in a children's classic, *The Secret Garden* (by Frances Hodgson Burnett). Colin, a sickly boy in a wheelchair, is slowly nurtured to health through the power of friendship and the exhilaration of coaxing a decrepit secret garden into beautiful bloom.

It appears that the mind can also *cause* illness. A couple of decades ago, two researchers at Rockefeller University performed some ground-breaking research. They repeatedly fed rats saccharin water, followed by an injection of a drug that made the rats sick. They then switched the drug to a harmless substance, but the rats still got sick. In other words, their minds were so conditioned that they got sick without exposure to the drug.

Many parents, when they first come to see me, are convinced that medication and supplements are the most important part of my program, and that everything else is secondary. Part of my job is to get across the idea that no one area of my Breath of Life asthma-prevention program is more important than another. In particular, I emphasize that one of a child's most potent weapons against asthma is her mind.

Don't assume that meditation and similar exercises are over your child's head. Indeed, when I teach the Breath of Life program, it is immediately apparent how readily children take to mind-body techniques. It is remarkable how easily I am able to get kids to lie down and quietly visualize peaceful scenes for several minutes at a time. Afterward, I will ask children to draw their visualizations. The pictures are beautiful, of kids in pastures with trees, of sailing on the water, of butterflies and birds. They are able to make a true mind-body connection, to visualize something clean and pure, and realize that that's how their lungs should feel. The children I work with experience a certain exhilaration when they sense that they are gaining control, that they have power over their fear, and that they can overcome asthma.

The following Breath of Life mind-body skills are the same ones I've had so much success with. Some of the techniques overlap somewhat, and learning one helps to reinforce another. Some can be done at home; others require an experienced practitioner. One of them, or a combination, will work for you and your child. I encourage you to choose a time of day that you can devote to these lessons, and simply put it into your permanent schedule. Don't be discouraged if your child gets distracted. Different exercises work better for different age groups. It's important to keep on trying. Mind-body training is like physical training—it takes a lot of practice.

Your persistence will be rewarded. For one thing, you will help your child reduce any stress that is making her illness worse. You and your child—as a team—will learn how to eliminate panic and stay calm in the face of an asthma attack. Your child will learn that asthma does not have to control her life. She will be confident that she can cope with whatever asthma throws at her, whether it's a tightening of the chest or a scary trip to the emergency room. According to the research discussed below, she may even reduce the inflammation and congestion that is causing her asthma. It's not a moment too soon, in fact, to spin your child's fear and anxiety into self-confidence and power. Teaching children these techniques early in life gives them a tool that they can use throughout life to cope with asthma or other stresses.

Of course, occasionally a child is stressed about an issue that may require outside counseling or psychological guidance. If you think that is the case, don't hesitate to talk to your school counselor, a therapist, or a psychologist.

BEFORE YOU BEGIN

Choose a quiet room in the house, where you can dim the lights and where there's a place for your child to relax and lie back. Before you begin the exercise, you might want to read a story or have your child read a story to you. Essentially, you want your child to get into a positive, relaxed state of mind, to associate these sessions with happy images and good feelings. Throughout each of the following exercises, you can incorporate the breathing lessons described in Chapter 7.

MEDITATION

Meditation produces a state of profound relaxation while the mind is still awake and alert. The idea is to clear and refocus your mind. In 1968, Herbert Benson and his colleagues at Harvard Medical School found that meditation slowed the heart and breathing down, calmed the immune system, and increased alpha brain waves, which are associated with relaxation. Benson first investigated meditation when he went to study with Tibetan monks, who would sit in a room that was twenty or thirty degrees, each draped in a wet towel. Through the power of meditation, they were able to increase their body temperature to the point where steam rose off their bodies.

Meditation is used to treat high blood pressure, heart disease, stroke, migraine headaches, and even autoimmune diseases such as arthritis. I've found it to be extremely beneficial for asthmatics as well.

How to Do It

Teach your child to meditate on a light, a beeswax candle flame, a sports trophy, or even a picture on the wall while counting. Have your child breathe in for three and out for four, or count one (inhale), two (exhale), three (inhale), and so on up to ten, and then start again. Or you can repeat a favorite word, such as *relax*. It may take weeks or months before your child is really able to concentrate. It's important to meditate in a comfortable chair with hands resting in the lap, sitting cross-legged on a cushion on the floor, or even lying down. Start with just a few minutes a day and slowly increase to ten to twenty minutes.

VISUALIZATION

One step beyond meditation is *visualization,* when you focus on positive images while in a relaxed state. Visualization has been the subject of much research by NIH psychiatrist Gerald Epstein, author of *Healing into Immortality* (ACMI, 2000) and a longtime proponent of the practice. Other studies have supported the use of visualization for asthmatics. An interesting study from the Netherlands found that asthmatic adolescents who focused on positive images had fewer episodes of breathlessness than those who concentrated on negative imagery. Asthmatic children who underwent hypnosis and visualization for six months had lower blood levels of IgE, the immunoglobulin associated with allergic episodes. A 1984 study of children with a variety of illnesses, including asthma, found that 51 percent of the kids whose treatment included self-hypnosis, relaxation, and visualization had complete resolution of their symptoms, and most of the others had some improvement. They also found that they were able to teach these techniques to children as young as three years old.

How to Do It

Ask your child to sit or lie on his bed or on a mat on the floor. Start with simple breathing exercises for a minute or two, inhaling with big belly breaths and exhaling fully. Then guide him to imagine a relaxing and comforting image, like a little boat moving along the water. Do this for about three minutes until he's fully relaxed. Then have him sit up and draw the image that he visualized. Initially, you want a simple visualization to get him used to the process. Other simple visualizations include: throwing a Frisbee, playing tennis, flying, a seed being carried by the wind, clothes drying in the wind, the tides, gliding, parachutes, radio and television waves, yachts, and windmills.

Once he's comfortable with a simple visualization, move on to the next step. Ask your child to visualize himself as healthy, strong, and participating in all his favorite activities. Slowly and softly talk him through a scenario: "You're picking up the baseball bat, you're swinging it, you hit it, and the ball flies into the stands." He should see himself on top of the world.

The next level is to visualize scenes that may seem more unsettling. Ask him to picture his last asthma episode. Describe the episode for him in simple terms and then ask him to visualize himself in a calm, quiet, and peaceful setting just like one he's in now with his mom or dad. Remind him that he feels confident because he knows he's going to be okay. Confront him with different challenges, where he visualizes himself first in a difficult place, and then in a place where he feels more comfortable. This exercise is an important step toward helping him to feel in control.

Finally, with an older child, ask him to visualize an asthma attack and how his body can fight it. Explain some basic anatomy first, preferably with a book to show him what the lungs, diaphragm, bronchi, and alveoli look like. Point out, for instance, that a tube called the *trachea* runs from the back of his throat to his lungs and that cells from his immune system course through his body, protecting him. During the exercise, encourage him to enlist the power of his body to fight asthma: "These are the tubes in your lungs; picture them opening. These are the cells of your immune system that help you to fight against infection. Picture these cells destroying anything that you breathe in that makes you feel bad." Tell him to picture himself surrounded by a white, warm healing force emanating from his hand. The feeling you want to get across is similar to the comfort of drinking the first sip of warm soup on a cold day. Tell him that he has the strength within himself to get through the difficult moments.

At each step, you can remind your child that you will be there to help him. You want to create a situation in which your child is going to trust you and know that you are fully engaged in this experience.

SELF-HYPNOSIS

People tend to be frightened of hypnosis and all the myths and mysticism around it. Don't be. Hypnosis can be a powerful tool to alleviate stress, and it can include autosuggestions that reprogram the mind and body. Researchers from the University of Minnesota found that hypnosis reduced doctor visits and that patients reported increased confidence in self-management skills. Under hypnosis, certain individuals have been able to produce anesthesia in different parts of their body. In fact, when injured or in shock from extreme stress, we instantly enter a kind of hypnotic state where things such as our movements, metabolisms, and respiratory rates are slowed. This is especially useful for older children.

How to Do It

It's important to learn hypnosis under the care of a physician who is familiar with this technique, though you can learn to do it at home with your child, and, ultimately, your child may learn to do self-hypnosis. Prior to beginning the session, you and your child can agree upon the signal to end the session, such as counting to three. Then have your child sit in a comfortable position in a chair, with her legs uncrossed. Place a beeswax candle before her and ask her to observe the flame. Or ask her to focus on a particular item in the room, like a book or your hand. As she observes it, suggest to her that her eyelids feel heavy, heavy enough to close. As she closes them, say a relaxing word, such as *relax* or *peace,* in cycles of three.

As she begins to breathe deeply and slowly, ask her to tighten and relax each area of her body. You can start with her toes, working up through her body, and ending by asking her to scrunch up her face and then relax it. As she continues to breathe deeply, tell her that she feels weighed down by a comfortable heavy weight, like a heavy blanket in a soft, warm bed. Continue to tell her that she is feeling really heavy and tired. As you count back from ten to zero, you can now encourage your child to breathe deeply and relax even more in between each count. All the while, her eyes should be closed. Let her know that she is in a state of complete relaxation and that her eyes should remain closed.

You can now give her certain positive suggestions, such as "Your lungs are being healed. Breathing is becoming easier and easier. You are not wheezing; your lungs are opening up. They are being bathed in soothing white light. Pure, healing oxygen is filling every part of your lungs. Each cell is being healed completely." When you wake her up, she'll feel refreshed and will remember all of your suggestions.

YOGA

Yoga combines proper breathing with relaxing postures that increase circulation, flexibility, and strength. According to studies published in the *Journal of Asthma,* yoga can significantly improve asthma symptoms. Researchers found that 66 percent of all patients were able to stop or reduce medications. Other studies have produced similar results. University students with asthma who practiced yoga reported much more relaxation, more positive attitudes, and less need of inhalers.

The most common type of yoga is *hatha yoga,* which focuses on breathing and stretching. *Kundalini yoga* involves breathing and chanting in an attempt to circulate energy from the base of the spine throughout the body. Simple yoga is not difficult to learn, and inexpensive classes are usually available at your local Y or gym. You and your child can start by getting an instructional video and practicing yoga in your living room.

Keep in mind that not all breathing exercises in yoga are appropriate for asthma, especially those that focus on breathing in rather than breathing out. Speak with your yoga instructor or doctor to make sure you're not doing these exercises.

BIOFEEDBACK

The science of biofeedback continues to improve. During biofeedback, doctors use sophisticated machines that help you to both monitor and become more aware of your body's internal processes. Biofeedback allows us to tune in to the involuntary ebb and flow of muscle tension, heart rate, blood pressure, brain wave activity, and skin temperature, among others. During biofeedback we learn to detect the subtle signals of stress, which can then allow us to make behavior modifications that can bring those abnormal readings back in line.

Biofeedback is a particularly good treatment for stress-related illnesses. It has even been used to help epileptics control seizures and to help cancer patients boost their immune systems. A June 2000 study found a decrease, as compared with a control group, in the severity of asthma symptoms in a group of non-steroid-dependent asthmatics who relied on biofeedback. *The Journal of Behavioral Medicine* recently reported that patients with a variety of conditions had a significant decrease in white blood cell counts while undergoing biofeedback training.

There are several different computer programs that can measure various vital signs, including rate of breathing, body temperature, rate of perspiration, and brain waves. There are also devices that are available for consumers, and although these are less sophisticated, they certainly may be quite helpful. If you do opt for biofeedback with a practitioner, the following will be evaluated:

- **Electromyogram (EMG):** Measures muscle tension, especially in your head and shoulders, where most of us tense up when under stress.
- **Temperature:** Records fluctuations in body temperature with a heat sensor on the hands, feet and fingers. Skin temperature lowers when we are anxious, and the idea here is to get yourself to raise your body temperature to lower the stress.
- **Galvanic Skin Response (GSR):** A dermograph measures electrical impulses in your skin. The lower the voltage, the more relaxed you are.
- **Electroencephalogram (EEG):** One of the most common biofeedback methods, an EEG images brain waves. When your brain emits alpha-level waves, you are in a relaxed state.

COGNITIVE REFRAMING

Reframing is useful in conjunction with the other techniques that we discuss in this chapter. Throughout many of the exercises discussed above, you may want to employ cognitive reframing to change your child's attitude toward asthma from one of frustration to one of freedom. The more confident he is when suffering asthmatic symptoms, the less likely he is to panic. Researchers at the University of Chicago found that people who viewed stress as a challenge and an opportunity had little physical reaction to stress. People who viewed their stress as uncontrollable and a threat had more illnesses.

How to Do It

Initially, you need to do this in a calm setting. Later on, your child can employ cognitive reframing anywhere, but first he must learn it without other distractions. The idea is to help your child put things in a more positive light. If he's constantly putting himself down, or you notice he's saying things that are discouraging, encourage him to take charge of his asthma in his own mind. Instead of saying, "I'm never going to get well. I'm never going to play hockey. I'm never going to be like everyone else," help him to think, "I am going to get better. I am going to play whatever sport I want to. I'm going to be able to do whatever I want."

During more advanced visualization and hypnosis sessions, you can help him learn to respond to flare-ups in a calm manner. First, ask him to remember a recent episode step by step and to visualize what his traditional, fearful response was. Then ask him to substitute one of the powerful methods discussed above in place of that fearful response. By putting in motion a series of steps that he's practiced, he can cope with the attack, and perhaps even prevent it from becoming serious.

If he had a bad event recently, for instance, ask him to step back and remember it. Maybe he was sitting in his friend's bedroom, and he reached out to pet his friend's cat. Suddenly he became short of breath and got very sick and scared. Go through it with him again, and reframe it by changing the ending. "You're uncomfortable and having trouble breathing. You check to see what might be causing those symptoms. You realize that it's the cat, and you leave the room. Instead of panicking, you relax and visualize your lungs opening up." Remind him that he has the tools to deal with asthma and the ability to reframe the story with a new, happy ending. The body remembers the last thing it did, and if he sits down and takes a moment to reframe the event with a better ending, his body stays with that thought.

A four-year-old girl came in last week. When drawing blood, I used something called a *butterfly needle.* As I was getting ready, I told her over and over that the needle was the butterfly and that it had a little sharp part, but once we put the butterfly in, she'd see a little of her blood come through the tube, and it would be red and pretty, and we'd use that blood to make sure that she stays healthy. She listened and watched, and while I was drawing blood she repeated almost verbatim, "Oh, that's the butterfly. Oh, there's the blood, and it's so pretty and red. It will make me stay healthy." Just this simple exercise made this four-year-old forget she was getting stuck with a needle.

ACUPUNCTURE AND KIDS

Acupuncture is an ancient mind-body treatment. It took a while for Western medicine to recognize the benefits of acupuncture, but the World Health Organization now lists acupuncture as one of the treatments for asthma. I have found acupuncture to be very helpful with my patients.

It is a system of medicine that is based on the belief that energy, or *chi,* flows through the body and can have a profound effect on health. Chi courses through energy channels in the body that are quite distinct from blood vessels or lymph vessels. When chi becomes blocked, energy becomes concentrated in the wrong place and, like a pool of water eroding a galvanized steel pipe, causes illness or unpleasant symptoms. Using needles that are inserted in acupuncture points, an acupuncturist *unclogs* the energy channel and normalizes the flow of chi. *The Journal of Traditional Chinese Medicine* ran a study that found that asthma patients were able to reduce their oral steroids significantly after thirty sessions of acupuncture over three months.

The practice of acupuncture is thousands of years old, one of the oldest treatments in the world. Legend has it that the practice has its roots in the story of a soldier who was wounded in battle by an arrow piercing his shoulder. It was noted that even though the soldier was injured, his asthma improved. Further experimentation revealed several points in the body that are linked to certain organ systems.

Surprisingly, many kids respond well to the idea of acupuncture, especially children who are old enough to understand what we're doing. For children who are less than enthusiastic about all those needles, parents can be taught *acupressure,* in which the fingers or hands are used instead of needles.

Acupuncture does require an expert practitioner. Check your local state acupuncture certifying board or www.drcity.com to find a local certified medical doctor.

OSTEOPATHIC MANIPULATION

As an osteopathic physician, I have found that children, especially older children, respond well to osteopathic manipulation. Through corrective thrusts or motions, an osteopath can realign and relax tissues or bones, allowing the body's immune system and other processes to return to normal. For asthma, this usually involves manipulation with one hand on either side of the spine, which may have been moved out of position due to the stress from an asthmatic event or an unrelated injury. Realigning the spine can improve the functioning of the nervous system as well as the immune system. Or asthmatic patients may require osteopathic manipulation that relaxes tensed accessory muscles in the back or neck that result from weeks or months of labored breathing. Often this requires applying gentle force through the patient's elbows, with one hand gently cupping the area of the back or neck that is tense.

Other valuable techniques for asthmatics include lymphatic drainage and massage. Lymph channels, like the bloodstream, flow throughout the body and occasionally get blocked due to injury or illness. By applying pressure over the lymph channels that run throughout the chest and into neighboring vessels, an osteopath can clear lymph channels and help improve the impaired immune system of an asthmatic.

For information about companion tapes on breathing and visualization, check the Dr City Health Store at www.drcity.com.

chapter nine

All in the Family

The first time a child comes into my office, I see a certain innocence in her eyes. What may seem like a standard process for most adults can be terrifying for children. A parent who understands the steps that need to be taken in a doctor's office can begin to smooth the way for their children. Understanding this and the myriad other family dynamics that asthma creates can help parents and siblings adapt to having a child with asthma in the family.

More work needs to be done to understand better the effects of asthma on children's psychological health. A recent study showed that children with mild to moderate asthma will probably suffer no long-term psychological consequences. This may be the case, but researchers still haven't even identified all the parameters that need to be measured when trying to quantify a child's happiness (to talk to other parents of asthmatic children, visit the Chat Room at www.drcity.com).

Few doctors or parents would dispute, however, that severe asthma presents many daily fears and frustrations, which, if not addressed, can lead to long-term psychological complications. When asthma is diagnosed, the parent and the child soon realize that this is the first of many visits to the asthma doctor. Your child may find that she cannot have a pet, or that a favorite sport may be difficult for her. At some point she may begin to focus on things she can't do, rather than things she can. These daily anxieties can put your child at risk for a lifetime of emotional distress and distrust. It's important to face this fact head-on and to understand that having an asthmatic child is going to alter your life considerably. Ideally, with the help of the Breath of Life program, those concerns and problems can be minimized.

Other relationships can also suffer from having a chronically ill child in the house. Sometimes asthmatic children require more attention than other children, resulting in resentment and jealousy. Sick children can also strain marriages, which can become particularly problematic when parents disagree over treatment.

One particular couple comes to mind. Sarah and Paul are divorced and had significant disagreements over the best approach for treating their child's asthma. Sarah wanted to use natural approaches; Paul wanted to focus on drugs. It became very tense in my office at times, and the child would act out by becoming distracted and disruptive, causing one or the other parent to snap at him and each other. Paul wanted his son to be a real boy, involved in sports and the owner of a dog. Sarah knew that these situations exacerbated her son's asthma. Paul was very distrustful of natural approaches, such as breathing exercises and supplements; Sarah, on the other hand, was probably too overprotective and overbearing when it came to her son playing sports and would not even consider using medication.

When the child would visit one parent, the other parent would later find out that all his or her directives weren't followed and would blame the subsequent flare-up on the ex-spouse.

I did finally convince the couple to go for family counseling. And even though there were issues that they couldn't resolve in their marriage, they were able to sit down for the sake of their child. We convinced Paul to hold off on getting a dog and to be more cautious about athletic activities. Sarah was able to give her son more leeway, to let her son be more involved in sports and understand the need for occasional medications. Even in this difficult situation, we were able to find room to cooperate for the sake of the child. There was a noticeable difference not only in the child's overall health but also in his confidence and in their support.

The final section of the Breath of Life program outlines strategies that will help your family halt the psychological damage that can develop if asthma escalates out of control. These guidelines come out of years of practicing with families who have had to cope with chronic illness in their midst. Of course, if the situation is intolerable or isn't getting better, professional counseling is advised. But most families, if they are willing to work together as a team, already have the power to stop this cycle of illness and despair. If everyone in the household is supportive and knowledgeable about the Breath of Life asthma program, your child will be buoyed by your love. This support can reduce, if not prevent, long-lasting psychological damage from asthma.

RECOGNIZE THAT YOUR CHILD IS AT RISK FOR DEPRESSION

Asthma is scary for children, not just because they have trouble breathing. It's scary because they learn to be afraid of their environment. It's scary because they sense parental fear. Generally children think their parents are invincible. They never question the fact that you will provide a roof over their heads, transportation, and food on the table. But when a child is struggling to breathe and his parents can't help him, he senses a breakdown in that structure. When a child sees that a parent is not confident in the face of asthma, he loses confidence too.

Studies have shown that asthmatics are more likely to be depressed and, later in life, tend to respond to stress more negatively. When something bad happens, asthmatics who are not adjusted to stresses in their life don't bounce back as easily as others. This fits in with a pattern of suffering that they've come to expect. One group of behavioral scientists compared a group of rats that had been treated well with a group of rats that had been abused. When they were placed in a water tank, the rats that were treated well would swim around in the water for hours, apparently convinced that they would be rescued. The abused rats would give up almost at once and drown.

Young adults with a history of asthma perceive stressful situations more often than people with no history of asthma. A study in *The Journal of Asthma* found that in southwestern Sydney, Australia, where there is a high rate of asthma, patients reported feeling lonely more often than their healthy peers. Another study in the same journal found that asthmatic children scored much higher in depression and lower on self-esteem than children with diabetes or cancer.

If you recognize early signs of depression—listlessness, acting withdrawn, and loss of appetite—the steps that follow may help.

Your child is also at risk for excess stress. An uptick in symptoms might be due to anxiety from a difficult teacher, tension between parents, or social issues like making the traveling soccer team. Kids pick up on a lot more than they let on. I'm always amazed when they come into my office and start to play on the floor, pull paper from the desk, and hide behind the furniture, all the while seemingly oblivious to my discussion with their parents. Then they come up with a question that shows they heard every word.

GET THE FAMILY INVOLVED

Fighting asthma takes the cooperation of many people in your child's life. If everyone is included, everyone is more motivated to help. Ideally, both parents will come to the first doctor's visits, or at least both parents should have a joint meeting with the doctor to fully discuss the asthma. In family strategy sessions, it's important to explain that this is just something that's a normal part of your family's life and that together you're going to have to make some adjustments. Encourage everyone to learn about the Breath of Life program to the best of his ability and to know that it is going to be stressful at times. It's important not to underestimate the effects of asthma. I always remind families that this can be a growing experience and that the information they learn can help all family members deal with stress and make them a healthier and happier family.

You should also help your family deal with the outside world. For every chronic illness, there are a million skeptics. Encourage everyone to be clear with friends and hard-nosed about issues like play dates and dietary restrictions, especially at parties and restaurants. Other parents and friends may need to be reminded again and again that asthma is not like strep throat. It doesn't go away after a few days. It's a confusing illness, because most of the time your child looks fine, but the truth is that asthma is an ongoing condition. You can't tell how an asthma patient is by how he or she looks on any given day.

HELP EVERYONE RECOGNIZE THAT A SICK CHILD MAY OCCASIONALLY NEED EXTRA ATTENTION

Certainly family dynamics can get out of whack when one child requires more time than the others. But with effort, it can be integrated into the normal family daily routines in a way that will minimize disruptions. If your child is waking up at night and can't breathe, and you are too tired the next day to take your other kids on a planned outing, certainly resentment can arise. One strategy is to assume that alternate *rain dates* should always be planned ahead of time, if possible. It helps to explain to the other kids that at this point in time, they may need to put some extra energy toward helping their asthmatic sibling get better. Enlist their help by telling them that you need their involvement. The goal here is to create an atmosphere that encourages everyone to realize that you're all in this together. Often, when both parents or the whole family consider themselves a part of the process, everyone ends up with a deeper commitment to the family's well-being.

HAVE REGULAR FAMILY MEETINGS

Families need to take extra time to talk to each other in order to lower anxiety and the deep sense of frustration that can sometimes occur when a family member has asthma. This can develop even after minor flare-ups, because of the enormous pressures that parents often find themselves under. A parent may be so consumed with the sick child that he or she may not notice signs of stress in another child before it's too late. If there's a built-in time to discuss concerns and make sure everyone is okay, this problem rarely arises.

The focus of these meetings is to establish a family-wide supportive and resilient attitude—that even though these situations are frightening, we can get through them. This is the time to air any grievances or complaints. It's also a good time to exchange information about asthma that your children probably don't know. You can encourage everyone to read about asthma and to make sure they all understand what all their options are. It's a good idea to have these meetings regularly, perhaps once a week for the first few weeks, and perhaps once a month thereafter.

This is also a time to set down policy and to give children information and direction. To minimize surprises later, explain in advance how things are going to be done.

Learn How to Resolve Conflicts

As with Sarah and Paul above, you may have one parent who believes only in traditional medicine and another who's committed to natural therapy. Generally, this becomes more of an issue if one or the other treatment fails and one parent wins out. Kids of divorced parents present even more problems, as there are now two households to detoxify and monitor and two parents who often have very different ideas about treatment. Grandparents and stepparents add even more layers of potential problems.

There are also unforeseen issues that you need to look at and honestly assess. Children pick up on stresses in marriages, or they may be anxious about a bully, or a certain activity at school. This increased stress just compounds their susceptibility to asthma attacks. You really need to take out the crystal ball and think about what's going on in the relationships between the parents, with children, with siblings, and with friends.

Conflict resolution involves establishing basic rules and agreeing to observe them. It's important that both parents know as much as possible about asthma. I find that arguments arise when one parent knows all the facts and the other is in the dark. First, you want to do whatever you can to reduce the risk of attack. Then follow up with rules that focus on getting your child healthy. Continue on this road until you get the desired result or until you've exhausted every possibility. Then it's back to the drawing board for another set of rules.

BE PREPARED FOR EMERGENCIES

You want to have a support system in place for emergencies. Not only will this reduce anxiety when there is an attack, but it will also say to your child that you're ready to help at any moment of the day.

In medical school, the first thing you are taught to do when you see someone who's in distress is to check your own pulse. Step one in an emergency for every parent is to stay calm, or your fear will be transferred to those around you and to your child. You also want to remember to be appropriately forceful and clear if you need help or are going to the emergency room.

Prepare an emergency center somewhere in the house, preferably by the kitchen phone. If and when an emergency occurs, you want to be able to take everything one step at a time; to be direct, clear, and to avoid panicking. Go over in your head and write down on paper instructions in case of an emergency: phone numbers of nearby friends, the local hospital, and your physician. Put these phone numbers by the phone or have them on speed dial. Know what to say immediately. Make sure you use the Breath of Life program to have a thorough understanding of your child's condition at all times.

Emergency treatment requires emergency medicine, and you should be very familiar with these drugs and how to administer them before an emergency begins. Write down information about administering medications. Start with the simplest, including use of an inhaler, a nebulizer, when to use an EpiPen, when to start cortisone, and when to call your doctor or go to an emergency room. Write down your doctor's specific recommendations—for instance, if your child wheezes for six hours, take x medication; for twelve hours, take y. Discuss this process with your physician to make sure you haven't missed anything.

If these steps are taken even in acute situations, a serious attack with long-term complications can be averted. I treated a seven-year-old girl named Megan whose asthma had been under control for three years. Then one Halloween she went to a friend's house and built a scarecrow stuffed with hay. The hay brought on a severe asthma attack. Even though it had been years since this had happened, her friend's mother called home and was given explicit instructions. Everyone knew what to do. Megan was removed from the area, the doctor was called, and Megan's mother quickly drove over with correct medications. This was done without panic, and Megan was soon feeling fine.

✂ How to Make Your Doctor Your Partner ✂

You want to find a doctor who's willing to listen and is open-minded about the many therapies and causes of asthma. You also need to connect with your asthma doctor. One style of practicing medicine may suit you and another may not—neither of which may have anything to do with the ability of the physician to provide care. If necessary, you may need to seek the guidance of an allergy specialist or a pulmonary specialist.

If a natural approach is what you want, make sure you get a doctor who's knowledgeable in the areas of nutrition, supplements, acupuncture, Oriental medicine, visualization, and biofeedback. It's important to choose the right doctor for your child's asthma, and to have a primary care physician who can coordinate your child's care. Finally, the better informed you are as a parent, the more you'll get out of your visits and the more normal your child's life will be. It's important to understand that your doctor is providing you with the best of his or her advice, and that the ideal situation is to create a trusting partnership.

FACE FACTS AND REAP THE BENEFITS

Many times parents come to see me bewildered that their child's asthma hasn't abated as quickly as they would have liked. I ask them if they've followed all my instructions, and invariably they say, "Yes, I've done *everything!*" Then I start to ask specific questions, and it comes out that there are no mattress covers on the beds, or the cat is still sleeping with the child, or the carpet hasn't yet been removed. Put bluntly, you must take inventory of your environment and your lifestyle, and make the changes that are necessary to eliminate the causes of your child's asthma. Have your checklist, go through it step by step, and be done with it.

And remember that there are some upsides to asthma, although these may be difficult to see at the time of an attack. Asthma teaches resilience and patience. Many asthmatics find themselves drawn to challenges and ultimately accomplish a great deal. Witness the triumphs of Olympic gold medalist Jackie Joyner-Kersee, who has battled asthma all her life. Following the Breath of Life program allows you to do something wonderful for your child—to help him get healthy. We have more technology and information than ever before on how to treat and prevent asthma, and with perseverance and effort, your child can live a healthy, normal, and active life. For more information about the Breath of Life program and the Firshein Center, please call 1–888–FIRSHEIN.

references

Chapter Two

Ball, T. M., Castro-Rodriguez, J. A., Griffith, K. A., Holberg, C. J., Martinez, F. D., & Wright, A. L. (2000). "Siblings, day-care attendance, and the risk of asthma and wheezing during childhood." *The New England Journal of Medicine* 343(8): 538–43.

Goldsmith, C. A., & Kobzik, L. (1999). "Particulate air pollution and asthma: A review of epidemiological and biological studies." *Reviews on Environmental Health* 14(3): 121–34.

Platts-Mills, T. A., Rakes, G., & Heymann, P. W. (2000). "The relevance of allergen exposure to the development of asthma in childhood." *The Journal of Allergy and Clinical Immunology* 105(2 Pt 2): S503–S508.

Sears, M. R., Burrows, B., Flannery, E. M., Herbison, G. P., Hewitt, C. J., & Holdaway, M. D. (1991). "Relation between airway responsiveness and serum IgE in children with asthma and in apparently normal children." *The New England Journal of Medicine* 325(15): 1067–71.

References

The International Study of Asthma and Allergies in Childhood (ISAAC) Steering Committee. (1998). "Worldwide variation in prevalence of symptoms of asthma, allergic rhinoconjunctivitis, and atopic eczema: ISAAC." *Lancet* 351(9111): 1225–32.

Additional Studies

Daugbjerg, P. (1989). "Is particle board in the home detrimental to health?" *Environmental Research* 48(2): 154–63.

Ezeamuzie, C. I., Thomson, M. S., Al-Ali, S., Dowaisan, A., Khan, M., & Hijazi, Z. (2000). "Asthma in the desert: Spectrum of the sensitizing aeroallergens." *Allergy* 55(2): 157–62.

Fauroux, B., Sampil, M., Quenel, P., & Lemoullec, Y. (2000). "Ozone: A trigger for hospital pediatric asthma emergency room visits." *Pediatric Pulmonology* 30(1): 41–46.

Garrett, M. H., Hooper, M. A., Hooper, B. M., Rayment, P. R., & Abramson, M. J. (1999). "Increased risk of allergy in children due to formaldehyde exposure in homes." *Allergy* 54(4): 330–37.

Gielen, M. H., van der Zee, S. C., van Wijnen, J. H., van Steen, C. J., & Brunekreef, B. (1997). "Acute effects of summer air pollution on respiratory health of asthmatic children." *American Journal of Respiratory and Critical Care Medicine* 155(6): 2105–8.

Hartert, T. V., & Peebles, R. S., Jr. (2000). "Epidemiology of asthma: The year in review." *Current Opinion in Pulmonary Medicine* 6(1): 4–9.

Hijazi, N., Abalkhail, B., & Seaton, A. (2000). "Diet and childhood asthma in a society in transition: A study in urban and rural Saudi Arabia." *Thorax* 55(9): 775–79.

Krieger, P., de Blay, F., Pauli, G., & Kopferschmitt, M. C. (1998). [Asthma and household chemical pollutants (with the exception of tobacco).] "Asthme et polluants chimiques domestiques (a l'exception du tabac)." *Revue des Maladies Respiratoires* 15(1): 11–24.

References

Krzyzanowski, M., Quackenboss, J. J., & Lebowitz, M. D. (1990). "Chronic respiratory effects of indoor formaldehyde exposure." *Environmental Research* 52(2): 117–25.

Linaker, C. H., Chauhan, A. J., Inskip, H. M., Holgate, S. T., & Coggon, D. (2000). "Personal exposures of children to nitrogen dioxide relative to concentrations in outdoor air." *Occupational and Environmental Medicine* 57(7): 472–76.

Mathison, D. A., Stevenson, D. D., & Simon, R. A. (1985). "Precipitating factors in asthma: Aspirin, sulfites, and other drugs and chemicals." *Chest* 87(1 Suppl): 50S–54S.

Meza, C., & Gershwin, M. E. (1997). "Why is asthma becoming more of a problem?" *Current Opinion in Pulmonary Medicine* 3(1): 6–9.

Nelson, H. S. (2000). "The importance of allergens in the development of asthma and the persistence of symptoms." *The Journal of Allergy and Clinical Immunology* 105(6 Pt 2): S628–S632.

Newson, R., Strachan, D., Archibald, E., Emberlin, J., Hardaker, P., & Collier, C. (1998). "Acute asthma epidemics, weather and pollen in England, 1987–1994." *European Respiratory Journal* 11(3): 694–701.

Nja, F., Roksund, O. D., Svidal, B., Nystad, W., & Carlsen, K. H. (2000). "Asthma and allergy among schoolchildren in a mountainous, dry, non-polluted area in Norway." *Pediatric Allergy and Immunology* 11(1): 40–48.

Perzanowski, M. S., Ronmark, E., Nold, B., Lundback, B., & Platts-Mills, T. A. (1999). "Relevance of allergens from cats and dogs to asthma in the northernmost province of Sweden: Schools as a major site of exposure." *The Journal of Allergy and Clinical Immunology* 103(6): 1018–24.

Romieu, I., Meneses, F., Ruiz, S., Sienra, J. J., Huerta, J., White, M. C., & Etzel, R. A. (1996). "Effects of air pollution on the respiratory health of asthmatic children living in Mexico City." *American Journal of Respiratory and Critical Care Medicine* 154(2 Pt 1): 300–7.

❧   References   ❧

Schwartz, J., Slater, D., Larson, T. V., Pierson, W. E., & Koenig, J. Q. (1993). "Particulate air pollution and hospital emergency room visits for asthma in Seattle." *The American Review of Respiratory Disease* 147(4): 826–31.

Thurston, G. D., Lippmann, M., Scott, M. B., & Fine, J. M. (1997). "Summertime haze air pollution and children with asthma." *American Journal of Respiratory and Critical Care Medicine* 155(2): 654–60.

Timonen, K. L., & Pekkanen, J. (1997). "Air pollution and respiratory health among children with asthmatic or cough symptoms." *American Journal of Respiratory and Critical Care Medicine* 156(2 Pt 1): 546–52.

Tolbert, P. E., Mulholland, J. A., MacIntosh, D. L., Xu, F., Daniels, D., Devine, O. J., Carlin, B. P., Klein, M., Dorley, J., Butler, A. J., Nordenberg, D. F., Frumkin, H., Ryan, P. B., & White, M. C. (2000). "Air quality and pediatric emergency room visits for asthma in Atlanta, Georgia, USA." *American Journal of Epidemiology* 151(8): 798–810.

Tseng, R. Y. & Li, C. K. (1990). "Low level atmospheric sulfur dioxide pollution and childhood asthma." *Annals of Allergy, Asthma and Immunology* 65(5): 379–83.

Varner, A. E., Busse, W. W., & Lemanske, R. F., Jr. (1998). "Hypothesis: Decreased use of pediatric aspirin has contributed to the increasing prevalence of childhood asthma." *Annals of Allergy, Asthma and Immunology* 81(4): 347–51.

von Mutius, E. (1996). "Progression of allergy and asthma through childhood to adolescence." *Thorax* 51(Suppl 1): S3–S6.

Weiss, S. T. (1997). "Diet as a risk factor for asthma." *Ciba Foundation Symposium* 206: 244–57, discussion 253–57.

Asthma Mortality
Chang, C. C., Phinney, S. D., Halpern, G. M., & Gershwin, M. E. (1993). "Asthma mortality: Another opinion—Is it a matter of life and . . . bread?" *Journal of Asthma* 30(2): 93–103.

Hannaway, P. J. (2000). "Demographic characteristics of patients experiencing near-fatal and fatal asthma: Results of a regional survey of 400 asthma specialists." *Annals of Allergy, Asthma and Immunology* 84(6): 587–93.

Hartert, T. V., & Peebles, R. S., Jr. (2000). "Epidemiology of asthma: The year in review." *Current Opinion in Pulmonary Medicine* 6(1): 4–9.

Chapter Three

Eggleston, P. A., & Wood, R. A. (1992). "Management of allergies to animals." *Allergy Proceedings* 13(6): 289–92.

Hodson, T., Custovic, A., Simpson, A., Chapman, M., Woodcock, A., & Green, R. (1999). "Washing the dog reduces dog allergen levels, but the dog needs to be washed twice a week." *The Journal of Allergy and Clinical Immunology* 103(4): 581–85.

Jaakkola, J. J., Verkasalo, P. K., & Jaakkola, N. (2000). "Plastic wall materials in the home and respiratory health in young children." *American Journal of Public Health* 90(5): 797–9.

Molfino, N. A., Wright, S. C., Katz, I., Tarlo, S., Silverman, F., McClean, P. A., Szalai, J. P., Raizenne, M., Slutsky, A. S., & Zamel, N. (1991). "Effect of low concentrations of ozone on inhaled allergen responses in asthmatic subjects." *Lancet* 338(8761): 199–203.

Nelson, H. S. (2000). "The importance of allergens in the development of asthma and the persistence of symptoms." *The Journal of Allergy and Clinical Immunology* 105(6 Pt 2): S628–S632.

Rosenstreich, D. L., Eggleston, P., Kattan, M., Baker, D., Slavin, R. G., Gergen, P., Mitchell, H., McNiff-Mortimer, K., Lynn, H., Ownby, D., & Malveaux, F. (1997). "The role of cockroach allergy and exposure to cockroach allergen in causing morbidity among inner-city children with asthma." *The New England Journal of Medicine* 336(19): 1356–63.

Vanlaar, C. H., Peat, J. K., Marks, G. B., Rimmer, J., & Tovey, E. R. (2000). "Domestic control of house dust mite allergen in children's beds." *The Journal of Allergy and Clinical Immunology* 105(6 Pt 1): 1130–33.

Wieslander, G., Norback, D., Walinder, R., Erwall, C., & Venge, P. (1999). "Inflammation markers in nasal lavage, and nasal symptoms in relation to relocation to a newly painted building: A longitudinal study." *International Archives of Occupational and Environmental Health* 72(8): 507–15.

Additional Studies
Abraham, M.E. (1999). "Microanalysis of indoor aerosols and the impact of a compact high-efficiency particulate air (HEPA) filter system." *Indoor Air* 9(1): 33–40.

Almqvist, C., Larsson, P. H., Egmar, A. C., Hedren, M., Malmberg, P., & Wickman, M. (1999). "School as a risk environment for children allergic to cats and a site for transfer of cat allergen to homes [see comments]." *The Journal of Allergy and Clinical Immunology* 103(6): 1012–17.

Carswell, F., Oliver, J., & Weeks, J. (1999). "Do mite avoidance measures affect mite and cat airborne allergens?" *Clinical and Experimental Allergy* 29(2): 193–200.

Dharmage, S., Bailey, M., Raven, J., Cheng, A., Rolland, J., Thien, F., Forbes, A., Abramson, M., & Walters, E. H. (1999). "Residential characteristics influence Der p 1 levels in homes in Melbourne, Australia." *Clinical and Experimental Allergy* 29(4): 461–69.

Eggleston, P. A., Rosenstreich, D., Lynn, H., Gergen, P., Baker, D., Kattan, M., Mortimer, K. M., Mitchell, H., Ownby, D., Slavin, R., & Malveaux, F. (1998). "Relationship of indoor allergen exposure to skin test sensitivity in inner-city children with asthma." *The Journal of Allergy and Clinical Immunology* 102(4 Pt 1): 563–70.

Hill, D. J., Thompson, P. J., Stewart, G. A., Carlin, J. B., Nolan, T. M., Kemp, A. S., & Hosking, C. S. (1997). "The Melbourne house dust mite study: Eliminating house dust mites in the domestic environment." *The Journal of Allergy and Clinical Immunology* 99(3): 3230.

Jalaludin, B., Xuan, W., Mahmic, A., Peat, J., Tovey, E., & Leeder, S. (1998). "Association between der p 1 concentration and peak expiratory flow rate in children with wheeze: A longitudinal analysis." *The Journal of Allergy and Clinical Immunology* 102(3): 382–86.

Mahmic, A., Tovey, E. R., Molloy, C. A., & Young, L. (1998). "House dust mite allergen exposure in infancy." *Clinical and Experimental Allergy* 28(12): 1487–92.

Moody, A., Fergusson, W., Wells, A., Bartley, J., & Kolbe, J. (2000). "Increased nitric oxide production in the respiratory tract in asymptomatic Pacific islanders: An association with skin prick reactivity to house dust mite." *The Journal of Allergy and Clinical Immunology* 105(5): 895–99.

Mosbech, H., Korsgaard, J., & Lind, P. (1988). "Control of house dust mites by electrical heating blankets." *The Journal of Allergy and Clinical Immunology* 81(4): 706–10.

Perzanowski, M. S., Ronmark, E., Nold, B., Lundback, B., & Platts-Mills, T. A. (1999). "Relevance of allergens from cats and dogs to asthma in the northernmost province of Sweden: Schools as a major site of exposure." *The Journal of Allergy and Clinical Immunology* 103(6): 1018–24.

Rains, N., Siebers, R., Crane, J., & Fitzharris, P. (1999). "House dust mite allergen (der p 1) accumulation on new synthetic and feather pillows." *Clinical and Experimental Allergy* 29(2): 182–85.

Reisman, R. E., Mauriello, P. M., Davis, G. B., Georgitis, J. W., & DeMasi, J. M. (1990). "A double-blind study of the effectiveness of a high-efficiency particulate air (HEPA) filter in the treatment of patients with perennial allergic rhinitis and asthma [see comments]." *The Journal of Allergy and Clinical Immunology* 85(6): 1050–57.

Sporik, R., Platts-Mills, T. A., & Cogswell, J. J. (1993). Exposure to house dust mite allergen of children admitted to hospital with asthma. *Clinical and Experimental Allergy* 23(9): 740–46.

van der Heide, S., van Aalderen, W. M., Kauffman, H. F., Dubois, A. E., & de Monchy, J. G. (1999). "Clinical effects of air cleaners in homes of asthmatic children sensitized to pet allergens." *The Journal of Allergy and Clinical Immunology* 104(2 Pt 1): 447–51.

Vanlaar, C. H., Peat, J. K., Marks, G. B., Rimmer, J., & Tovey, E. R. (2000). "Domestic control of house dust mite allergen in children's beds." *The Journal of Allergy and Clinical Immunology* 105(6 Pt 1): 1130–33.

Vaughan, J. W., McLaughlin, T. E., Perzanowski, M. S., & Platts-Mills, T. A. (1999). "Evaluation of materials used for bedding encasement: Effect of pore size in blocking cat and dust mite allergen." *The Journal of Allergy and Clinical Immunology* 103(2 Pt 1): 227–31.

Vichyanond, P., Uthaisangsook, S., Ruangruk, S., & Malainual, N. (1999). "Complete mattress encasing is not superior to partial encasing in the reduction of mite allergen." *Allergy* 54(7): 736–41.

Warner, J. A., Frederick, J. M., Bryant, T. N., Weich, C., Raw, G. J., Hunter, C., Stephen, F. R., McIntyre, D. A., & Warner, J. O. (2000). "Mechanical ventilation and high-efficiency vacuum cleaning: A combined strategy of mite and mite allergen reduction in the control of mite-sensitive asthma." *The Journal of Allergy and Clinical Immunology* 105(1 Pt 1): 75–82.

Weeks, J., Oliver, J., Birmingham, K., Crewes, A., & Carswell, F. (1995). "A combined approach to reduce mite allergen in the bedroom." *Clinical and Experimental Allergy* 25(12): 1179–83.

Chapter Four

Forastiere, F., Pistelli, R., Sestini, P., Fortes, C., Renzoni, E., Rusconi, F., Dell'Orco, V., Ciccone, G., & Bisanti, L. (2000). "Consumption of fresh fruit rich in vitamin C and wheezing symptoms in children. SIDRIA Collaborative Group, Italy (Italian Studies on Respiratory Disorders in Children and the Environment)." *Thorax* 55(4): 283–88.

McNeal, James. *The Kids' Market: Myths and Realities* (Ithaca: Paramount Market Publishing Inc., 1999).

Seaton, A., & Devereux, G. (2000). "Diet, infection and wheezy illness: Lessons from adults." *Pediatric Allergy and Immunology* 11(Suppl 13): 37–40.

Additional Studies

Chang, C. C., Phinney, S. D., Halpern, G. M., & Gershwin, M. E. (1993). "Asthma mortality: Another opinion—Is it a matter of life and . . . bread?" *Journal of Asthma* 30(2): 93–103.

Hijazi, N., Abalkhail, B., & Seaton, A. (2000). "Diet and childhood asthma in a society in transition: A study in urban and rural Saudi Arabia." *Thorax* 55(9): 775–79.

Weiss, S. T. (1997). "Diet as a risk factor for asthma." *Ciba Foundation Symposium*, 206, 244–57, discussion 253–57.

Chapter Five

Agertoft, L., & Pedersen, S. (2000). "Effect of long-term treatment with inhaled budesonide on adult height in children with asthma." *The New England Journal of Medicine* 343(15): 1064–69.

Bisgaard, H., Loland, L., & Oj, J. A. (1999). "No in exhaled air of asthmatic children is reduced by the leukotriene receptor antagonist montelukast." *American Journal of Respiratory and Critical Care Medicine* 160(4): 1227–31.

Garbe, E., Suissa, S., & LeLorier, J. (1998). "Association of inhaled corticosteroid use with cataract extraction in elderly patients" [published erratum appears in *JAMA* 280(21): 1830]. *The Journal of the American Medical Association* 280(6): 539–43.

Kennedy, W. A., Laurier, C., Gautrin, D., Ghezzo, H., Pare, M., Malo, J. L., & Contandriopoulos, A. P. (2000). "Occurrence and risk factors of oral candidiasis treated with oral antifungals in seniors using inhaled steroids." *Journal of Clinical Epidemiology* 53(7): 696–701.

La Revue Prescrire. (2000). "Montelukast. No current use for asthma." *Canadian Family Physician* 46(1): 86–99.

Lipworth, B. J. (1999). "Systemic adverse effects of inhaled corticosteroid therapy: A systematic review and meta-analysis." *Archives of Internal Medicine* 159(9): 941–55.

Malinverni, R., Kuo, C. C., Campbell, L. A., & Grayston, J. T. (1995). "Reactivation of Chlamydia pneumoniae lung infection in mice by cortisone." *The Journal of Infectious Diseases* 172(2): 593–94.

Mitchell, P., Cumming, R. G., & Mackey, D. A. (1999). "Inhaled corticosteroids, family history, and risk of glaucoma." *Ophthalmology* 106(12): 2301–6.

Plotnick, L. H., & Ducharme, F. M. (2000). "Combined inhaled anticholinergic agents and beta-2-agonists for initial treatment of acute asthma in children." *Cochrane Database of Systematic Reviews* (2), CD000060.

Reicin, A., White, R., Weinstein, S. F., Finn, A. F., Jr., Nguyen, H., Peszek, I., Geissler, L., & Seidenberg, B. C. (2000). "Montelukast, a leukotriene receptor antagonist, in combination with loratadine, a histamine receptor antagonist, in the treatment of chronic asthma." *Archives of Internal Medicine* 160(16): 2481–88.

Sharek, P. J., & Bergman, D. A. (2000). "The effect of inhaled steroids on the linear growth of children with asthma: A meta-analysis." *Pediatrics* 106(1): E8.

Skoner, D. P., Szefler, S. J., Welch, M., Walton-Bowen, K., Cruz-Rivera, M., & Smith, J. A. (2000). "Longitudinal growth in infants and young children treated with budesonide inhalation suspension for persistent asthma." *The Journal of Allergy and Clinical Immunology* 105(2 Pt 1): 259–68.

The Childhood Asthma Management Program Research Group. (2000). "Long-term effects of budesonide or nedocromil in children with asthma." *The New England Journal of Medicine* 343(15): 1054–63.

Wong, C. A., Walsh, L. J., Smith, C. J., Wisniewski, A. F., Lewis, S. A., Hubbard, R., Cawte, S., Green, D. J., Pringle, M., & Tattersfield, A. E. (2000). "Inhaled corticosteroid use and bone-mineral density in patients with asthma." *Lancet* 355(9213): 1399–1403.

Yoshida, S., Amayasu, H., Sakamoto, H., Onuma, K., Shoji, T., Nakagawa, H., & Tajima, T. (1998). "Cromolyn sodium prevents bronchoconstriction and urinary LTE4 excretion in aspirin-induced asthma." *Annals of Allergy, Asthma and Immunology* 80(2): 171–76.

Additional Studies

Bisgaard, H. (2000). "Long-acting beta-2-agonists in management of childhood asthma: A critical review of the literature [see comments]." *Pediatric Pulmonology* 29(3): 221–34.

Byrnes, C., Shrewsbury, S., Barnes, P. J., & Bush, A. (2000). "Salmeterol in pediatric asthma." *Thorax* 55(9): 780–84.

Crowley, S., Hindmarsh, P. C., Matthews, D. R., & Brook, C. G. (1995). "Growth and the growth hormone axis in prepubertal children with asthma." *The Journal of Pediatrics* 126(2): 297–303.

Diaz, T., Sturm, T., Matte, T., Bindra, M., Lawler, K., Findley, S., & Maylahn, C. (2000). "Medication use among children with asthma in East Harlem." *Pediatrics* 105(6): 1188–93.

Dickinson, E. T., O'Connor, R. E., & Megargel, R. (1992). "The prehospital use of nebulized albuterol on patients with wheezing whose chief complaint is shortness of breath." *Delaware Medical Journal* 64(11): 679–83.

DiGiulio, G. A., Kercsmar, C. M., Krug, S. E., Alpert, S. E., & Marx, C. M. (1993). "Hospital treatment of asthma: Lack of benefit from theophylline given in addition to nebulized albuterol and intravenously administered corticosteroids." *The Journal of Pediatrics* 122(3): 464–69.

Edwards, A. M., Lyons, J., Weinberg, E., Weinberg, F., Gillies, J. D., Reid, G., Robertson, C. F., Robinson, P., Dalton, M., Van Asperen, P., Wilson, C., Mullineux, J., Mullineux, A., Sly, P. D., Cox, M., & Isles, A. F. (1999). "Early use of inhaled nedocromil sodium in children following an acute episode of asthma." *Thorax* 54(4): 308–15.

Gries, D. M., Moffitt, D. R., Pulos, E., & Carter, E. R. (2000). "A single dose of intramuscularly administered dexamethasone acetate is as effective as oral prednisone to treat asthma exacerbations in young children." *The Journal of Pediatrics* 136(3): 298–303.

Gutglass, D. J., Hampers, L., Roosevelt, G., Teoh, D., Nimmagadda, S. R., & Krug, S. E. (2000). "Undiluted albuterol aerosols in the pediatric emergency department." *Pediatrics* 105(5): E67.

Kannisto, S., Korppi, M., Remes, K., & Voutilainen, R. (2000). "Adrenal suppression, evaluated by a low dose adrenocorticotropin test, and growth in asthmatic children treated with inhaled steroids." *The Journal of Clinical Endocrinology and Metabolism* 85(2): 652–57.

Korhonen, K., Korppi, M., Remes, S. T., Reijonen, T. M., & Remes, K. (1999). "Lung function in school-aged asthmatic children with inhaled cromoglycate, nedocromil and corticosteroid therapy." *The European Respiratory Journal* 13(1): 82–86.

Mathison, D. A., Stevenson, D. D., & Simon, R. A. (1985). "Precipitating factors in asthma. Aspirin, sulfites, and other drugs and chemicals." *Chest* 87(1 Suppl): 50S–54S.

Pradalier, A., & Vincent, D. (2000). "Aspirine: Allergie ou intolerance. [Aspirin: Allergy or intolerance.]" *La Revue de Medecine Interne* 21(Suppl 1): 75S–82S.

Qureshi, F., Pestian, J., Davis, P., & Zaritsky, A. (1998). "Effect of nebulized ipratropium on the hospitalization rates of children with asthma." *The New England Journal of Medicine* 339(15): 1030–35.

Schuh, S., Parkin, P., Rajan, A., Canny, G., Healy, R., Rieder, M., Tan, Y. K., Levison, H., & Soldin, S. J. (1989). "High-versus low-dose, frequently administered, nebulized albuterol in children with severe, acute asthma." *Pediatrics* 83(4): 513–18.

Schuh, S., Reider, M. J., Canny, G., Pender, E., Forbes, T., Tan, Y. K., Bailey, D., & Levison, H. (1990). Nebulized albuterol in acute childhood asthma: comparison of two doses. *Pediatrics* 86(4): 509–13.

Schuh, S., Reisman, J., Alshehri, M., Dupuis, A., Corey, M., Arseneault, R., Alothman, G., Tennis, O., & Canny, G. (2000). "A comparison of inhaled fluticasone and oral prednisone for children with severe acute asthma." *The New England Journal of Medicine* 343(10): 689–94.

Sekerel, B. E., Saraclar, Y., Etikan, I., & Kalayci, O. (1999). "Comparison of two different dose regimens of nedocromil sodium with placebo in the management of childhood asthma." *Journal of Investigational Allergology and Clinical Immunology* 9(5): 293–98.

Shaheen, S. O., Sterne, J. A., Songhurst, C. E., & Burney, P. G. (2000). "Frequent paracetamol use and asthma in adults." *Thorax* 55(4): 266–70.

Warner, J. O. (1989). "The place of Intal in paediatric practice." *Respiratory Medicine* 83(Suppl): 33–37.

Wolfe, J., Rooklin, A., Grady, J., Munk, Z. M., Stevens, A., Prillaman, B., Duke, S., & Harding, S. (2000). "Comparison of once- and twice-daily dosing of fluticasone propionate 200 micrograms per day administered by diskus device in patients with asthma treated with or without inhaled corticosteroids." *The Journal of Allergy and Clinical Immunology* 105(6 Pt 1): 1153–61.

Chapter Six
Albanes, D., Heinonen, O. P., Taylor, P. R., Virtamo, J., Edwards, B. K., Rautalahti, M., Hartman, A. M., Palmgren, J., Freedman, L. S., Haapakoski, J., Barrett, M. J., Pietinen, P., Malila, N., Tala, E., Liippo, K., Salomaa, E. R., Tangrea, J. A., Teppo, L., Askin, F. B., Taskinen, E., Erozan, Y., Greenwald, P., & Huttunen, J. K. (1996). "Alpha-Tocopherol and beta-carotene supplements and lung cancer incidence in the alpha-tocopherol, beta-carotene cancer prevention study: Effects of base-line characteristics and study compliance." *Journal of the National Cancer Institute* 88(21): 1560–70.

Baker, J. C., Tunnicliffe, W. S., Duncanson, R. C., & Ayres, J. G. (1999). "Dietary antioxidants and magnesium in type 1 brittle asthma: A case control study." *Thorax* 54(2): 115–18.

Bielory, L., & Gandhi, R. (1994). "Asthma and vitamin C." *Annals of Allergy* 73(2): 89–96.

Bilimoria, M. H., & Ecobichon, D. J. (1992). "Protective antioxidant mechanisms in rat and guinea pig tissues challenged by acute exposure to cigarette smoke." *Toxicology* 72(2): 131–44.

Broughton, K. S., Johnson, C. S., Pace, B. K., Liebman, M., & Kleppinger, K. M. (1997). "Reduced asthma symptoms with n-3 fatty acid ingestion are related to 5-series leukotriene production." *The American Journal of Clinical Nutrition* 65(4): 1011–17.

Busse, W. W., Kopp, D. E., & Middleton, E., Jr. (1984). "Flavonoid modulation of human neutrophil function." *The Journal of Allergy and Clinical Immunology* 73(6): 801–809.

Emelyanov, A., Fedoseev, G., & Barnes, P. J. (1999). "Reduced intracellular magnesium concentrations in asthmatic patients." *The European Respiratory Journal* 13(1): 38–40.

Flatt, A., Pearce, N., Thomson, C. D., Sears, M. R., Robinson, M. F., & Beasley, R. (1990). "Reduced selenium in asthmatic subjects in New Zealand." *Thorax* 45(2): 95–99.

Fox, C. H., Ramsoomair, D., Mahoney, M. C., Carter, C., Young, B., & Graham, R. (1999). "An investigation of hypomagnesemia among ambulatory urban African-Americans." *Journal of Family Practice* 48(8): 636–39.

Hasselmark, L., Malmgren, R., Zetterstrom, O., & Unge, G. (1993). "Selenium supplementation in intrinsic asthma." *Allergy* 48(1): 30–36.

Kadrabova, J., Mad'aric, A., Podivinsky, F., Gazdik, F., & Ginter, F. (1996). "Plasma zinc, copper and copper/zinc ratio in intrinsic asthma." *Journal of Trace Elements in Medicine and Biology* 10(1): 50–53.

Kelly, F. J. (1999). "Glutathione: In defense of the lung." *Food and Chemical Toxicology* 37(9–10): 963–66.

Kelly, F. J., Mudway, I., Blomberg, A., Frew, A., & Sandstrom, T. (1999). "Altered lung antioxidant status in patients with mild asthma [letter]." *Lancet* 354(9177): 482–83.

Malvy, D. J., Burtschy, B., Arnaud, J., Sommelet, D., Leverger, G., Dostalova, L., Drucker, J., & Amedee-Manesme, O. (1993). "Serum beta-carotene and antioxidant micronutrients in children with cancer. The 'Cancer in Children and Antioxidant Micronutrients' French Study Group." *International Journal of Epidemiology* 22(5): 761–71.

Mangat, H. S., D'Souza, G. A., & Jacob, M. S. (1998). "Nebulized magnesium sulphate versus nebulized salbutamol in acute bronchial asthma: A clinical trial." *The European Respiratory Journal* 12(2): 341–44.

Mossad, S. B., Macknin, M. L., Medendorp, S. V., & Mason, P. (1996). "Zinc gluconate lozenges for treating the common cold. A randomized, double-blind, placebo-controlled study [see comments]." *Annals of Internal Medicine* 125(2): 81–88.

Pearce, F. L., Befus, A. D., & Bienenstock, J. (1984). "Mucosal mast cells III. Effect of quercetin and other flavonoids on antigen-induced histamine secretion from rat intestinal mast cells." *The Journal of Allergy and Clinical Immunology* 73(6): 819–23.

Pryor, W. A., Stahl, W., & Rock, C. L. (2000). "Beta carotene: From biochemistry to clinical trials." *Nutrition Reviews* 58(2 Pt 1): 39–53.

Rowe, B. H., Bretzlaff, J. A., Bourdon, C., Bota, G. W., & Camargo, C. A., Jr. (2000). "Magnesium sulfate for treating exacerbations of acute asthma in the emergency department." *Cochrane Database of Systematic Reviews* (2): CD001490.

Schwartz, J. (2000). "Role of polyunsaturated fatty acids in lung disease." *The American Journal of Clinical Nutrition* 71(1 Suppl): 393S–396S.

Soutar, A., Seaton, A., & Brown, K. (1997). "Bronchial reactivity and dietary antioxidants." *Thorax* 52(2): 166–70.

⁊ References ⁊

Tekin, D., Sin, B. A., Mungan, D., Misirligil, Z., & Yavuzer, S. (2000). "The antioxidative defense in asthma." *Journal of Asthma,* 37(1): 59–63.

van der Put, N. M., Steegers-Theunissen, R. P., Frosst, P., Trijbels, F. J., Eskes, T. K., van den Heuvel, L. P., Mariman, E. C., den Heyer, M., Rozen, R., & Blom, H. J. (1995). "Mutated methylenetetrahydrofolate reductase as a risk factor for spina bifida." *Lancet* 346(8982): 1070–71.

Additional Studies
Boner, A. L., Valletta, E. A., Andreoli, A., Vallone, G., & Baronio, L. (1984). "A combination of cefuroxime and N-acetyl-cysteine for the treatment of maxillary sinusitis in children with respiratory allergy." *International Journal of Clinical Pharmacology, Therapy, and Toxicology* 22(9): 511–14.

Ciarallo, L., Sauer, A. H., & Shannon, M. W. (1996). "Intravenous magnesium therapy for moderate to severe pediatric asthma: Results of a randomized, placebo-controlled trial." *The Journal of Pediatrics* 129(6): 809–14.

Dominguez, L. J., Barbagallo, M., Di Lorenzo, G., Drago, A., Scola, S., Morici, G., & Caruso, C. (1998). "Bronchial reactivity and intracellular magnesium: A possible mechanism for the bronchodilating effects of magnesium in asthma." *Clinical Science* (Colch) 95(2): 137–42.

Fogarty, A., & Britton, J. (2000). "Nutritional issues and asthma." *Current Opinion in Pulmonary Medicine* 6(1): 86–89.

Hatch, G. E. (1995). "Asthma, inhaled oxidants, and dietary antioxidants." *The American Journal of Clinical Nutrition* 61(3 Suppl): 625S–630S.

Kalayci, O., Besler, T., Kilinc, K., Sekerel, B. E., & Saraclar, Y. (2000). "Serum levels of antioxidant vitamins (alpha tocopherol, beta carotene, and ascorbic acid) in children with bronchial asthma." *Turkish Journal of Pediatrics* 42(1): 17–21.

Li, M. H., Zhang, H. L., & Yang, B. Y. (1997). [Effects of ginkgo leave concentrated oral liquor in treating asthma.] *Zhongguo Zhong Xi Yi Jie He Za Zhi* 17(4): 216–18 (Chinese).

Neuman, I., Nahum, H., & Ben-Amotz, A. (1999). "Prevention of exercise-induced asthma by a natural isomer mixture of beta-carotene." *Annals of Allergy, Asthma and Immunology* 82(6): 549–53.

Pennings, H. J., Borm, P. J., Evelo, C. T., & Wouters, E. F. (1999). "Changes in levels of catalase and glutathione in erythrocytes of patients with stable asthma, treated with beclomethasone dipropionate." *The European Respiratory Journal* 13(6): 1260–66.

Reynolds, R. D., & Natta, C. L. (1985). "Depressed plasma pyridoxal phosphate concentrations in adult asthmatics." *The American Journal of Clinical Nutrition* 41(4): 684–88.

Chapter Seven
Ben-Zvi, Z., Spohn, W. A., Young, S. H., & Kattan, M. (1982). "Hypnosis for exercise-induced asthma." *The American Review of Respiratory Disease* 125(4): 392–95.

Bingol Karakoc, G., Yilmaz, M., Sur, S., Ufuk Altintas, D., Sarpel, T., & Guneter Kendirli, S. (2000). "The effects of daily pulmonary rehabilitation program at home on childhood asthma." *Allergologia et Immunopathologia* 28(1): 12–14.

Field, T., Henteleff, T., Hernandez-Reif, M., Martinez, E., Mavunda, K., Kuhn, C., & Schanberg, S. (1998). "Children with asthma have improved pulmonary functions after massage therapy." *The Journal of Pediatrics* 132(5): 854–58.

Hackman, R. M., Stern, J. S., & Gershwin, M. E. (2000). "Hypnosis and asthma: A critical review." *The Journal of Asthma* 37(1): 1–15.

Hunt, J., & Gaston, B. (2000). "Airway nitrogen oxide measurements in asthma and other pediatric respiratory diseases." *The Journal of Pediatrics* 137(1): 14–20.

Chapter Eight
Benson, H., Malhotra, M. S., Goldman, R. F., Jacobs, G. D., & Hopkins, P. J. (1990). "Three case reports of the metabolic and electroencephalographic changes during advanced Buddhist meditation techniques." *Behavioral Medicine* 16(2): 90–95.

References

Erskine-Milliss, J., & Schonell, M. (1981). "Relaxation therapy in asthma: A critical review." *Psychosomatic Medicine* 43(4): 365–72.

Hu, J. (1998). "Clinical observation on 25 cases of hormone dependent bronchial asthma treated by acupuncture." *Journal of Traditional Chinese Medicine* 18(1): 27–30.

Kohen, D. P., & Wynne, E. (1997). "Applying hypnosis in a preschool family asthma education program: Uses of storytelling, imagery, and relaxation." *American Journal of Clinical Hypnosis* 39(3): 169–81.

Kohen, D. P., Olness, K. N., Colwell, S. O., & Heimel, A. (1984). "The use of relaxation-mental imagery (self-hypnosis) in the management of 505 pediatric behavioral encounters." *Journal of Developmental and Behavioral Pediatrics* 5(1): 21–25.

McGrady, A., Conran, P., Dickey, D., Garman, D., Farris, E., & Schumann-Brzezinski, C. (1992). "The effects of biofeedback-assisted relaxation on cell-mediated immunity, cortisol, and white blood cell count in healthy adult subjects." *Journal of Behavioral Medicine* 15(4): 343–54.

Nagendra, H. R., & Nagarathna, R. (1986). "An integrated approach of yoga therapy for bronchial asthma: A 3–54-month prospective study." *The Journal of Asthma* 23(3): 123–37.

Scherr, M. S., & Crawford, P. L. (1978). Three-year evaluation of biofeedback techniques in the treatment of children with chronic asthma in a summer camp environment. *Annals of Allergy* 41(5): 288–92.

Vedanthan, P. K., Kesavalu, L. N., Murthy, K. C., Duvall, K., Hall, M. J., Baker, S., & Nagarathna, S. (1998). "Clinical study of yoga techniques in university students with asthma: A controlled study." *Allergy and Asthma Proceedings* 19(1): 3–9.

Zanus, L., Cracco, A., Mesirca, P., & Ronconi, G. F. (1984). Il biofeedback nel bambino asmatico. [Biofeedback in asthmatic children.] *La Pediatria Medica e Chirurgica* 6(2): 247–51.

Chapter Nine

Bender, B. G., Annett, R. D., Ikle, D., DuHamel, T. R., Rand, C., & Strunk, R. C. (2000). "Relationship between disease and psychological adaptation in children in the Childhood Asthma Management Program and their families. CAMP Research Group." *Archives of Pediatrics and Adolescent Medicine* 154(7): 706–13.

Forero, R., Bauman, A., Young, L., Booth, M., & Nutbeam, D. (1996). "Asthma, health behaviors, social adjustment, and psychosomatic symptoms in adolescence." *Journal of Asthma* 33(3): 157–64.

Mullins, L. L., Chaney, J. M., Pace, T. M., Hartman, V. L. (1997). "Illness uncertainty, attributional style, and psychological adjustment in older adolescents and young adults with asthma." *Journal of Pediatric Psychology* 22(6): 871–80.

index

Index

Dr. Richard N. Firshein is a leading authority in the field of preventive medicine and medical nutrition and Medical Director of the Firshein Center for Comprehensive Medicine in New York City. Board certified in family medicine and a certified medical acupuncturist, he is the author of two groundbreaking books, *Reversing Asthma* and *The Nutraceutical Revolution,* and creator of the Breath of Life Asthma Prevention Program. His practice specializes in integrative medicine, developing comprehensive programs for a wide range of conditions, including asthma and allergies. These comprehensive programs combine nutritional supplementation, personal diets, and body-mind therapies, as well as traditional medical approaches.

Faced with the challenge of asthma early in his own life, Dr. Firshein developed the Breath of Life program detailed here, which he uses in his practice for all age groups. As Medical Director of the Sorvino Asthma Foundation, Dr. Firshein, along with Paul Sorvino, was honored for their work with asthmatic children. Dr. Firshein has served as a professor of family medicine at the New York College of Osteopathic Medicine. For more information about Dr. Firshein and his work, visit the Web site, www.drcity.com, or call his office directly at 1–888–FIRSHEIN.